BREAST FEEDING SECRETS REVEALED

QUEEN WILZ

COPYWRITE AND LEGAL DISCLAIMER:

The information contained in this book is for general informational purposes only. While every effort has been made to ensure the accuracy and completeness of the information provided, the author and publisher make no representations or warranties of any kind, express or implied, about the completeness, accuracy, reliability, suitability, or availability with respect to the contents of this book for any purpose. The information is provided on an "as is" basis.

The author and publisher do not provide medical advice. The content of this book is not intended to be a substitute for professional medical advice, diagnosis, or treatment. Always seek the advice of your physician or other qualified health provider with any questions you may have regarding a medical condition. Never disregard professional medical advice or delay in seeking it because of something you have read in this book.

The author and publisher disclaim any liability or responsibility for any loss, injury, or damage incurred as a consequence, directly or indirectly, of the use and application of any of the contents of this book.

Any reliance you place on the information contained in this book is strictly at your own risk. The author and publisher shall not be liable for any direct, indirect, incidental, consequential, or special damages arising out of the use of or inability to use this book or any information contained herein, even if advised of the possibility of such damages.

All trademarks, product names, company names, logos, and other intellectual property referred to in this book are the property of their respective owners and are used for identification

purposes only. The use of such names does not imply any affiliation with or endorsement by the trademark owners.

By reading this book, you agree to abide by the terms and conditions set forth in this disclaimer. If you do not agree to these terms, you should not use this book. Your use of this book indicates your acceptance of these terms.

PREFACE

Welcome to "Breastfeeding Secrets Revealed"!

Dear Reader,
I am thrilled to introduce you to this transformative journey
into the world of breastfeeding. As a mother, a passionate
advocate for maternal health, and a dedicated researcher, it is
my honor to share with you the insights, wisdom, and secrets
that I have uncovered along the way.

Breastfeeding is a profound experience—a sacred bond that
connects mother and baby in ways that words alone cannot
capture. It is a journey of discovery, of joy, and of
empowerment—a journey that I am deeply passionate about
guiding you through.

In this book, you will discover a treasure trove of knowledge,
from the fundamentals of lactation to the intricacies of nursing
positions, from the challenges of early days to the triumphs of
long-term breastfeeding. I have poured my heart and soul into
these pages, distilling years of research, personal experience,
and the invaluable wisdom of countless mothers and experts.

But more than just a practical guide, "Breastfeeding Secrets
Revealed" is a celebration of the extraordinary power of
breastfeeding—a celebration of the strength and resilience of
mothers, the miraculous capabilities of the female body, and
the profound impact that breastfeeding has on the health and
well-being of both mother and child.

As you embark on this journey with me, I encourage you to approach it with an open heart and an open mind. Embrace the challenges, savor the triumphs, and above all, trust in yourself and in the incredible journey that lies ahead.

Thank you for entrusting me with your breastfeeding journey. It is my greatest hope that this book will serve as a source of inspiration, empowerment, and support as you embark on this beautiful and transformative chapter of motherhood.

With warmest regards,

Queen Wilz

COPYWRITE AND LEGAL DISCLAIMER: *2*

PREFACE *4*

INTRODUCTION: WELCOME TO THE JOURNEY OF BREASTFEEDING *7*

CHAPTER 1: UNDERSTANDING BREASTFEEDING BASICS *17*

CHAPTER 2: PREPARING FOR BREASTFEEDING *28*

CHAPTER 3: THE FIRST FEW DAYS *37*

CHAPTER 4: NUTRITION FOR NURSING MOTHERS *47*

CHAPTER 5: OVERCOMING COMMON BREASTFEEDING ISSUES *57*

CHAPTER 6: BREASTFEEDING TECHNIQUES AND TIPS *68*

CHAPTER 8: BREASTFEEDING IN PUBLIC *88*

CHAPTER 10: SPECIAL CIRCUMSTANCES *107*

CHAPTER 11: HEALTH AND WELLNESS *116*

CHAPTER 12: BUILDING A SUPPORT NETWORK *127*

CHAPTER 13: INSPIRATIONAL STORIES *141*

CONCLUSION: YOUR BREASTFEEDING JOURNEY AHEAD *151*

Welcome to "Breastfeeding Secrets Revealed." As you open the pages of this book, you are embarking on an extraordinary journey — one that is deeply personal, profoundly enriching, and incredibly rewarding. Breastfeeding is more than just a method of feeding your baby; it is a journey of love, connection, and nourishment that will shape the bond between you and your child in ways that are both beautiful and lasting.

I am Queen Wilz, and it is my honor to be your guide on this journey. As a mother who has navigated the ups and downs of breastfeeding and a nurse with years of experience in holistic wellness, I have witnessed firsthand the transformative power of breastfeeding. My own experiences, combined with the knowledge I have gained from helping countless mothers, have inspired me to write this book. I aim to share with you the secrets, insights, and practical advice that will empower you to breastfeed with confidence and joy.

Breastfeeding is a natural and instinctive process, yet it often comes with challenges and uncertainties. Many new mothers find themselves facing questions and concerns: Will my baby latch properly? Am I producing enough milk? How do I handle the discomfort? These are common worries, and this book is here to address them all, offering you the support and guidance you need to navigate each stage of your breastfeeding journey.

In "Breastfeeding Secrets Revealed," we will explore everything from the basics of breastfeeding anatomy to the intricacies of milk production, from the first latch to weaning, and from overcoming common challenges to balancing breastfeeding with the demands of daily life. Each chapter is filled with expert advice, practical tips, and inspirational stories from mothers who have been where you are now.

This book is not just a manual; it is a celebration of the incredible bond that breastfeeding creates. It is a testament to the strength, resilience, and love that define the experience of nurturing your baby. You will find that breastfeeding is not just about feeding your baby; it is about building a foundation of health, trust, and connection that will last a lifetime.

As you read through these pages, I encourage you to approach breastfeeding with an open heart and an open mind. Embrace the journey, with its joys and challenges, and know that you are not alone. You have a community of mothers, healthcare professionals, and supporters who are here to help you every step of the way.

Thank you for allowing me to be a part of your breastfeeding journey. Together, we will unlock the secrets to successful breastfeeding, ensuring that you and your baby enjoy this precious time to the fullest.

Welcome to the journey of breastfeeding. Let's begin this beautiful adventure together.

Warmly,
Queen Wilz.

A Warm Welcome: Introducing the Author and the Purpose of the Book

Welcome to "Breastfeeding Secrets Revealed"! I'm Queen Wilz, and I am thrilled to be your guide on this extraordinary journey. As a mother, nurse, and holistic wellness advocate, my passion for supporting mothers through the breastfeeding process comes from both professional experience and personal triumphs.

Breastfeeding is one of the most natural and profound ways to bond with and nourish your baby. Yet, as many new mothers discover, it is not always as straightforward as one might expect. There can be questions, challenges, and moments of doubt. It is my mission to provide you with the knowledge, encouragement, and practical tools to navigate these moments with confidence and grace.

My journey into the world of breastfeeding began with the birth of my first child. Like many of you, I faced my own set of challenges, from initial latching difficulties to balancing breastfeeding with the demands of daily life. Through perseverance, support, and a lot of learning, I discovered the incredible rewards that breastfeeding offers. This experience inspired me to help other mothers by sharing the insights I gained and the secrets I uncovered along the way.

"Breastfeeding Secrets Revealed" is more than just a guide — it's a comprehensive resource designed to support you at every stage of your breastfeeding journey. Whether you're preparing for your first breastfeeding experience, encountering unexpected hurdles, or looking to deepen your understanding of this incredible process, this book has something for you.

In these pages, you'll find detailed information about the anatomy of breastfeeding, practical tips for overcoming common challenges, and strategies for balancing breastfeeding with the demands of modern life. You'll learn about the nutritional needs of nursing mothers, techniques for increasing milk supply, and ways to ensure a successful return to work while continuing to breastfeed. Additionally, the book is filled with inspiring stories from other mothers who have faced and overcome their own breastfeeding challenges.

The purpose of this book is to empower you with the knowledge and confidence to make breastfeeding a fulfilling and successful experience. Each chapter is crafted to address real-life concerns and provide actionable advice, so you feel supported and informed every step of the way.

As you embark on this journey, remember that breastfeeding is a deeply personal experience. There is no one-size-fits-all approach, and what works for one mother and baby may not work for another. This book encourages you to find what works best for you and your baby, fostering a connection that is unique and beautiful.

Thank you for allowing me to be a part of your breastfeeding journey. Together, we will unlock the secrets to successful breastfeeding, ensuring that you and your baby enjoy this precious time to the fullest.

Welcome to the journey of breastfeeding. Let's embark on this beautiful adventure together.

Warm regards,

Queen Wilz.

The Power of Breastfeeding: Benefits for Both Mother and Baby

Breastfeeding is a remarkable and powerful act that provides numerous benefits for both mother and baby. It is a natural way to nourish your child, offering an unparalleled start in life. Beyond nutrition, breastfeeding fosters a deep emotional connection and contributes to the overall well-being of both mother and baby. Let's explore the profound benefits that breastfeeding brings to this unique and irreplaceable bond.

For the Baby:
Optimal Nutrition:
Breast milk is perfectly tailored to meet your baby's nutritional needs. It contains the right balance of proteins, fats, vitamins, and minerals, ensuring that your baby receives all the essential nutrients for healthy growth and development.

Immunity Boost:
Breast milk is rich in antibodies and immune-boosting elements that protect your baby from infections and illnesses. These antibodies help strengthen your baby's immune system, reducing the risk of respiratory infections, ear infections, and gastrointestinal issues.

Healthy Growth and Development:
Breastfed babies tend to have better physical and cognitive development. The unique composition of breast milk supports brain development, which can lead to higher IQ scores and improved cognitive function later in life.

Reduced Risk of Chronic Conditions:

Breastfeeding has been linked to a lower risk of developing chronic conditions such as asthma, allergies, obesity, and type 2 diabetes. It also reduces the risk of sudden infant death syndrome (SIDS).

Digestive Health:
Breast milk is easily digestible and promotes healthy gut flora, reducing the likelihood of constipation, colic, and other gastrointestinal issues.

For the mother:
Emotional Bonding:
Breastfeeding fosters a deep emotional connection between mother and baby. The skin-to-skin contact and the act of nursing release oxytocin, the "love hormone," which enhances bonding and emotional attachment.

Physical Health Benefits:
Breastfeeding helps the mother's body recover more quickly after childbirth. It promotes uterine contractions that reduce postpartum bleeding and help the uterus return to its pre-pregnancy size.

Weight Management:
Breastfeeding burns extra calories, which can help you return to your pre-pregnancy weight more quickly. It also helps in reshaping your body naturally.

Reduced Risk of Certain Cancers:
Studies have shown that breastfeeding lowers the risk of breast and ovarian cancers. The longer you breastfeed, the greater the protective effect.
Convenience and Cost Savings:

Breastfeeding is convenient and economical. There's no need to buy formula, prepare bottles, or sterilize equipment, making it easier to feed your baby on demand, anytime and anywhere.

Long-term Benefits:
Emotional and Psychological Well-being:
The strong bond formed through breastfeeding can have lasting positive effects on both mother and baby's emotional and psychological well-being. This bond fosters a sense of security and trust that benefits your child's emotional health well into adulthood.

Sustainable and Environmentally Friendly:
Breastfeeding is a natural, renewable resource that requires no packaging or transportation, reducing your environmental footprint and contributing to a more sustainable lifestyle.

Conclusion:
The power of breastfeeding extends far beyond providing nutrition. It is a profound act that nurtures, protects, and connects mother and baby in extraordinary ways. Embracing the journey of breastfeeding allows you to experience its full spectrum of benefits, creating a foundation of health, happiness, and emotional strength for both you and your baby.

As you embark on this incredible journey, remember that every drop of breast milk counts and every moment spent breastfeeding is a step towards a healthier and stronger future for you and your baby. Celebrate the power of breastfeeding and cherish the beautiful bond it creates.

Overcoming Myths: Addressing Common Misconceptions about Breastfeeding

Breastfeeding, despite being a natural and ancient practice, is surrounded by numerous myths and misconceptions. These misunderstandings can create unnecessary anxiety and barriers for new mothers. By addressing and debunking these myths, we can empower mothers with accurate information, helping them make informed decisions about breastfeeding. Here are some common misconceptions and the truths behind them:

Myth 1: "Breastfeeding is always painful."
Truth: While some discomfort is normal in the first few days, breastfeeding should not be painful. Pain usually indicates an issue, such as improper latch or positioning. With proper guidance and support, most mothers can breastfeed comfortably.

Myth 2: "You need to eat a perfect diet to produce quality milk."
Truth: A well-balanced diet is beneficial for your overall health, but your body will still produce nutritious milk even if your diet is not perfect. It is important to eat healthily, but occasional indulgences won't harm your breast milk.

Myth 3: "You can't breastfeed if you have small breasts."
Truth: Breast size does not determine milk production. Women with small breasts can produce just as much milk as those with larger breasts. Milk production is influenced by demand and supply mechanisms, not breast size.

Myth 4: "Formula is just as good as breast milk."
Truth: While formula can provide necessary nutrients, breast milk contains antibodies, live cells, and enzymes that formula cannot replicate. Breast milk is specifically tailored to your baby's needs and offers unmatched health benefits.

Breastfeeding is a natural and instinctive process, but it often comes with a learning curve for both mother and baby. Understanding the fundamentals of breastfeeding can set a strong foundation for a successful and enjoyable breastfeeding journey. This chapter will cover the essential basics, from the anatomy of lactation to the mechanics of a proper latch.

1.1 The Anatomy of Lactation
Understanding how your body produces and delivers milk is crucial for successful breastfeeding. Here are the key components involved:

Mammary Glands: These are specialized glands located within the breast tissue that produce milk.
Alveoli: Tiny milk-producing sacs within the mammary glands. When stimulated by hormones, they secrete milk.
Milk Ducts: These ducts transport milk from the alveoli to the nipple.
Nipple and Areola: The nipple is the protruding part from which milk is delivered, while the areola is the darker area surrounding the nipple. The baby latches onto the areola, not just the nipple, to nurse effectively.
1.2 The Hormones of Breastfeeding
Several hormones play a vital role in the production and release of breast milk:

Prolactin: This hormone stimulates the production of milk. Prolactin levels rise when your baby nurses or you pump milk.

Oxytocin: Known as the "love hormone," oxytocin causes the milk ejection reflex, also known as the let-down reflex, which releases milk from the alveoli into the milk ducts and out through the nipple.

Estrogen and Progesterone: These hormones prepare your breasts for milk production during pregnancy but drop significantly after birth to allow lactation to begin.

1.3 The Mechanics of a Proper Latch

A proper latch is critical for effective breastfeeding and to prevent nipple soreness. Here are the steps to achieve a good latch:

Positioning: Hold your baby close, with their belly facing yours. Support their head, neck, and shoulders.

Nipple Alignment: Touch your nipple to your baby's upper lip to encourage them to open their mouth wide.

Achieving the Latch: When your baby opens their mouth wide, bring them to your breast, ensuring they take in a large portion of the areola, not just the nipple.

Checking the Latch: Your baby's lips should be flanged outwards, and you should see more areola above their upper lip than below their lower lip. Their chin should touch your breast, and you should feel a deep, rhythmic suckling rather than sharp pain.

1.4 Understanding Feeding Cues

Recognizing when your baby is hungry can help you feed them before they become distressed. Common feeding cues include:

Early Cues: Rooting (turning head with mouth open), sucking on hands or fingers, and lip smacking.

Mid Cues: Increased physical activity, fussiness, and searching for the breast.

Late Cues: Crying and turning red. It's best to feed your baby before they reach this stage.

1.5 Establishing a Feeding Schedule
In the early weeks, feeding your baby on demand is crucial for establishing milk supply and ensuring they get enough to eat. Signs your baby is getting enough milk include:

Frequent Wet Diapers: At least six wet diapers a day after the first week.
Regular Bowel Movements: Several stools per day initially, which may decrease over time.
Steady Weight Gain: Regular weight checks with your pediatrician can confirm proper growth.
1.6 Common Challenges and Solutions

Every breastfeeding journey has its ups and downs. Here are some common challenges and tips for overcoming them:

Sore Nipples: Ensure a proper latch, use lanolin cream, and allow nipples to air dry.
Engorgement: Nurse frequently, apply warm compresses before feeding, and cold compresses afterward.
Low Milk Supply: Nurse or pump more often, stay hydrated, and consider lactation supplements after consulting with a healthcare provider.
Blocked Ducts: Massage the area, apply warm compresses, and continue nursing frequently.
Conclusion
Understanding the

basics of breastfeeding is the first step towards a successful and rewarding experience for both you and your baby. By familiarizing yourself with the anatomy and physiology of lactation, mastering the mechanics of a proper latch, recognizing feeding cues, establishing a feeding schedule, and knowing how to overcome common challenges, you can confidently embark on your breastfeeding journey. Remember, every mother and baby pair are unique, and what works for one may not work for another. Trust in your body's ability to nourish your baby and seek support when needed. This knowledge will empower you to provide the best possible start for your baby and create a strong, loving bond through breastfeeding.

Anatomy of Lactation: How Breastfeeding Works
Breastfeeding is a complex and finely tuned process that involves various parts of the female anatomy working together to produce and deliver milk to the baby. Understanding the anatomy of lactation can help you appreciate the miraculous process your body undergoes to nourish your child and troubleshoot any issues that may arise. Here's an in-depth look at how breastfeeding works:

The Breast Structure
The primary structures involved in lactation are the mammary glands, milk ducts, alveoli

Anatomy of Lactation: How Breastfeeding Works
Breastfeeding is a complex and finely tuned process that involves various parts of the female anatomy working together to produce and deliver milk to the baby. Understanding the anatomy of lactation can help you appreciate the miraculous process your body undergoes to nourish your child and troubleshoot any issues that may arise. Here's an in-depth look at how breastfeeding works:

The Breast Structure
The primary structures involved in lactation are the mammary glands, alveoli, milk ducts, and the nipple and areola. Each part plays a crucial role in the production and delivery of milk.

Mammary Glands: These are specialized organs within the breast that are responsible for producing milk. Each breast contains 15-20 lobes, and each lobe is made up of smaller lobules.

Alveoli: These are tiny, grape-like clusters of cells located within the lobules. The alveoli are the milk-producing units. They secrete milk into the small ducts that lead to larger ducts.

Milk Ducts: These ducts transport milk from the alveoli to the nipple. As the baby nurses, the milk ducts widen to facilitate the flow of milk. The ducts converge at the nipple, where milk is released during breastfeeding.

Nipple and Areola: The nipple is the protruding part from which milk is delivered. Surrounding the nipple is the areola, a darker area of skin that helps the baby locate the nipple. The areola contains glands that secrete an oily substance to keep the nipple moisturized and prevent cracking.

The Role of Hormones
Hormones play a pivotal role in regulating lactation. The primary hormones involved are prolactin and oxytocin.

Prolactin: This hormone is essential for milk production. When your baby sucks at the breast, it stimulates the pituitary gland in your brain to release prolactin. Prolactin signals the alveoli to produce milk. Higher levels of prolactin are produced at night, which is why nighttime feedings are important for maintaining milk supply.

Oxytocin: Known as the "love hormone," oxytocin is responsible for the milk ejection reflex, also known as the let-down reflex. When your baby begins to nurse, oxytocin causes the muscles around the alveoli to contract and push milk through the milk ducts to the nipple. Oxytocin also helps the uterus contract after childbirth, aiding in recovery.

The Milk Production Process
Milk production operates on a supply-and-demand basis. The more your baby nurses, the more milk your body will produce. This process can be broken down into several key steps:

Stimulation: When your baby latches onto your breast and begins to suckle, it stimulates the nerves in the nipple and areola.

Hormonal Response: This stimulation sends signals to your brain to release prolactin and oxytocin.

Milk Production: Prolactin signals the alveoli to produce milk.

Milk Ejection: Oxytocin causes the muscles around the alveoli to contract, pushing milk through the ducts to the nipple.

Nursing: Your baby's sucking and swallowing create a cycle that encourages continued milk production and ejection.

The Let-Down Reflex

The let-down reflex is crucial for breastfeeding success. It can be triggered by various stimuli, including your baby's cry, thoughts of your baby, or physical touch. Some mothers feel a tingling or warm sensation when let-down occurs, while others may not feel anything at all. Stress and anxiety can inhibit the let-down reflex, so it's important to create a calm and comfortable environment for breastfeeding.

Colostrum and Mature Milk
Colostrum: The first milk produced after childbirth is called colostrum. It is thick, yellowish, and packed with antibodies and nutrients that are vital for newborn health. Colostrum is produced in small amounts but is highly concentrated.

Transitional Milk: A few days after birth, colostrum transitions into mature milk. During this phase, the milk becomes thinner and increases in volume.

Mature Milk: Mature milk contains the perfect balance of nutrients, including fats, proteins, and carbohydrates, to support your baby's growth and development. It consists of foremilk, which is waterier and quenches your baby's thirst, and hindmilk, which is richer in fat and calories to satisfy hunger.

Conclusion
Understanding the anatomy of lactation helps demystify the breastfeeding process and empowers you to overcome potential challenges. By knowing how your body produces and delivers milk, you can better appreciate the natural ability to nourish your baby and address any issues that may arise with confidence.

Breastfeeding Positions: Finding What Works Best for You and Your Baby

Finding the right breastfeeding position is essential for both you and your baby's comfort and effectiveness of feeding. Each mother-baby pair is unique, so experimenting with different positions can help you discover what works best. Here's a guide to some of the most common breastfeeding positions, along with tips on how to use them effectively.

Cradle Hold

Description:

The cradle hold is one of the most traditional and widely used breastfeeding positions. In this position, you support your baby's head in the crook of your arm, with their body turned towards you.

How to:

Sit comfortably with good back support.
Hold your baby in your arm, with their head resting in the crook of your elbow on the same side you are nursing.
Align your baby's stomach with your stomach, and their mouth level with your nipple.
Use your other hand to support your breast if necessary.
Tips:

Use a pillow to support your arm and your baby's weight.
Ensure your baby's head and body are aligned to avoid neck strain.

Cross-Cradle Hold

Description:

The cross-cradle hold provides more control over your baby's head, making it easier to achieve a good latch, especially for newborns and premature babies.

How to:

Sit comfortably with a pillow supporting your back.
Hold your baby across your body with the opposite arm to the
breast you are feeding from (i.e., use your left arm to hold
your baby when nursing from the right breast).

Support your baby's head with your hand, placing your
thumb and fingers around their neck and head.
Use your other hand to support your breast and guide your
baby's mouth to your nipple.
Tips:

This position is particularly useful for mothers with small or
premature babies who need more head support.
Ensure your baby's head and body are well-aligned and close
to your breast.
Football Hold (Clutch Hold)
Description:
The football hold, also known as the clutch hold, is especially
helpful for mothers recovering from a cesarean section or
those with large breasts or twins.

How to:

Sit comfortably with good back support and a pillow at your
side.
Position your baby at your side, under your arm, with their
body facing you and their legs pointing towards your back.
Support your baby's head and neck with your hand, and use
your forearm to support their back.
Use your other hand to support your breast and guide your
baby to latch.

Tips:

This position keeps pressure off your abdomen, making it ideal post-cesarean.
Use a pillow to support your arm and keep your baby at breast height.
Side-Lying Position
Description:

The side-lying position is excellent for nighttime feedings or if you want to rest while nursing. It allows both you and your baby to lie down.

How to:

Lie on your side with a pillow under your head and another behind your back for support.
Place your baby on their side facing you, with their nose level with your nipple.
Use your lower arm to cradle your baby's back or head, and your upper arm to adjust your breast.
Tips:

Ensure your baby's mouth is aligned with your nipple.
Keep pillows and blankets away from your baby's face to avoid suffocation risks.
Laid-Back Position (Biological Nurturing)
Description:
The laid-back position encourages a natural breastfeeding experience, taking advantage of gravity to help your baby latch. It's also great for bonding and skin-to-skin contact.

How to:

Recline comfortably on a couch or bed, supported by pillows.

Place your baby on your chest, tummy down, allowing them to find your nipple naturally.
Use your hands to support your baby's back and head if needed.
Tips:

This position can help with issues like oversupply or a strong let-down reflex.
Relax and let your baby use their instincts to latch on.

Conclusion
Choosing the right breastfeeding position is crucial for a comfortable and successful breastfeeding journey. Each position offers unique benefits and can be suited to different stages and situations. Experiment with these positions to find what works best for you and your baby, ensuring that both of you are comfortable and relaxed during feedings. Remember, breastfeeding is a learning process, and finding the perfect position may take time and practice. Trust your instincts and seek support from lactation consultants if needed.

Chapter 2: Preparing for Breastfeeding

Breastfeeding success often begins before your baby arrives. Preparation is key to overcoming challenges and ensuring a smooth start to your breastfeeding journey. In this chapter, we will explore the essential steps to prepare for breastfeeding, from gathering knowledge and resources to setting up a supportive environment for you and your baby.

Gathering Knowledge: Understanding the basics of breastfeeding, including the benefits for both mother and baby, the mechanics of lactation, and common challenges, is crucial. Educate yourself by reading reputable sources, attending breastfeeding classes, and seeking guidance from healthcare professionals or lactation consultants.

Building a Support Network: Surround yourself with a supportive network of family, friends, and professionals who can offer encouragement, advice, and practical assistance. Joining breastfeeding support groups or online communities can also provide valuable peer support and guidance.

Choosing Healthcare Providers: Select healthcare providers who are knowledgeable and supportive of breastfeeding. Your obstetrician, pediatrician, and lactation consultant should be experienced in breastfeeding management and able to offer personalized guidance and support.

Preparing Your Body: Take steps to optimize your health and prepare your body for breastfeeding during pregnancy. Stay hydrated, eat a balanced diet rich in nutrients, and engage in gentle exercises to promote overall wellness. Discuss any concerns or medical conditions with your healthcare provider to address them proactively.

Assembling Breastfeeding Supplies: Stock up on essential breastfeeding supplies, including nursing bras, breast pads, nipple cream, and a breast pump if needed. Consider investing in a comfortable nursing pillow and breastfeeding-friendly clothing to enhance your comfort during feedings.

Creating a Breastfeeding-Friendly Environment: Designate a comfortable and private space in your home where you can breastfeed comfortably and without interruption. Ensure that you have a supportive chair or nursing station, adequate lighting, and all necessary supplies within reach.

Educating Your Support System: Educate your partner, family members, and caregivers about the importance of breastfeeding and how they can support you in your breastfeeding journey. Communicate your needs and preferences clearly, and enlist their help in managing household tasks and caring for your baby to allow you ample time for breastfeeding and rest.

Addressing Potential Challenges: Anticipate potential challenges that may arise during breastfeeding, such as latch difficulties, engorgement, or nipple pain, and familiarize yourself with strategies to overcome them. Having a plan in place can help you navigate challenges confidently and prevent them from derailing your breastfeeding goals.

By taking proactive steps to prepare for breastfeeding, you can set the stage for a successful and fulfilling breastfeeding experience for both you and your baby. Embrace the journey with confidence, knowing that you have equipped yourself with the knowledge, support, and resources needed to thrive as a breastfeeding mother.

Prenatal Preparation: Getting Ready Before Baby Arrives

Preparing for breastfeeding during pregnancy is an essential step in ensuring a smooth transition to breastfeeding after your baby is born. By taking proactive measures and gathering necessary resources beforehand, you can set yourself up for breastfeeding success. Here's a guide to prenatal preparation for breastfeeding:

Education and Information:

Educate yourself about the benefits of breastfeeding for both you and your baby. Understanding the advantages, such as immune system support, bonding, and optimal nutrition, can reinforce your commitment to breastfeeding.
Attend prenatal breastfeeding classes or workshops to learn about breastfeeding techniques, positioning, latch, and common challenges. These classes provide valuable knowledge and practical skills that will serve you well once your baby arrives.
Nutritional Preparation:

Focus on maintaining a healthy diet rich in nutrients during pregnancy to support optimal breastfeeding outcomes. Aim to consume a variety of fruits, vegetables, whole grains, lean proteins, and healthy fats to ensure that you and your baby receive essential nutrients.

Discuss any dietary concerns or nutritional needs with your healthcare provider, especially if you have specific dietary restrictions or medical conditions that may affect breastfeeding.
Breast Care:

Practice good breast hygiene and care during pregnancy to keep your breasts healthy and comfortable. Avoid using harsh soaps or lotions on your nipples and areolas, as these can cause dryness or irritation.
Consider using a lanolin-based nipple cream or coconut oil to moisturize your nipples and prevent cracking or soreness. Gentle massage and warm compresses can also help alleviate discomfort and promote circulation.
Setting Realistic Expectations:

Understand that breastfeeding may come with its challenges, especially in the early weeks. Setting realistic expectations and being prepared for potential difficulties can help you navigate any bumps in the road with confidence and resilience. Remember that every breastfeeding journey is unique, and it's okay to seek support and guidance when needed. Trust your instincts and be patient with yourself as you and your baby learn to breastfeed together.

Gathering Supplies:

Assemble essential breastfeeding supplies, such as nursing bras, breast pads, nipple cream, and a breast pump if you plan to express milk. Having these items on hand before your baby arrives can streamline the breastfeeding process and help you feel prepared.
Consider investing in a comfortable nursing chair or pillow to support your body during breastfeeding sessions. Having a designated breastfeeding area in your home can also create a peaceful and conducive environment for breastfeeding.

Support System:

Surround yourself with a supportive network of family, friends, and healthcare providers who are knowledgeable about breastfeeding and can offer encouragement and assistance. Communicate your breastfeeding goals and preferences with your support system to ensure they understand how best to support you.
By taking proactive steps to prepare for breastfeeding during pregnancy, you can set a strong foundation for a successful breastfeeding journey. With education, support, and preparation, you'll be well-equipped to nourish and nurture your baby through breastfeeding from the moment they arrive.

Essential Supplies: Must-Have Items for Successful Breastfeeding

Having the right supplies on hand can significantly enhance your breastfeeding experience and support your journey as a breastfeeding mother. Here are the essential supplies every breastfeeding mother should consider:

Nursing Bras:

Invest in comfortable and supportive nursing bras designed specifically for breastfeeding mothers. Nursing bras feature convenient clasps or panels that allow easy access for breastfeeding or pumping.
Breast Pads:

Breast pads, also known as nursing pads, help absorb leaks and prevent embarrassing stains on your clothing. Choose between disposable or reusable breast pads based on your preference and budget.
Nipple Cream:

Nipple cream or ointment can soothe sore or cracked nipples, providing relief and promoting healing. Look for lanolin-based creams or natural alternatives that are safe for both you and your baby.

Breast Pump:

A breast pump can be a valuable tool for breastfeeding mothers, allowing you to express milk for times when you're away from your baby or need to increase milk supply. Choose between manual or electric breast pumps based on your needs and preferences.

Milk Storage Containers:

Milk storage containers or bags are essential for storing expressed breast milk safely. Opt for BPA-free containers or bags that are designed specifically for breast milk storage and can be easily labeled and dated.

Nursing Pillow:

A nursing pillow provides support and comfort during breastfeeding sessions, helping you maintain proper positioning and reducing strain on your back and arms. Choose a nursing pillow with a firm yet comfortable design that fits your body shape.

Breastfeeding-Friendly Clothing:

Invest in breastfeeding-friendly clothing that allows easy acccss for nursing or pumping. Look for tops or dresses with discreet nursing openings or front panels that can be easily lifted or unbuttoned for breastfeeding.

Water Bottle:

Staying hydrated is essential for maintaining milk supply and overall health while breastfeeding. Keep a water bottle nearby during breastfeeding sessions to ensure you stay hydrated and replenish fluids lost during nursing.
Breastfeeding App or Journal:

Consider using a breastfeeding app or journal to track feeding sessions, diaper changes, and other important milestones. These tools can help you monitor your baby's feeding patterns and identify any issues that may arise.
Lactation Support:

Don't underestimate the value of professional lactation support. Consider enlisting the help of a lactation consultant or joining a breastfeeding support group to receive personalized guidance, troubleshooting tips, and encouragement on your breastfeeding journey.
By having these essential supplies on hand, you can feel confident and prepared to navigate the ups and downs of breastfeeding with ease and comfort. Remember that every breastfeeding journey is unique, so don't hesitate to seek support and guidance from healthcare professionals or fellow breastfeeding mothers as needed.

Creating a Supportive Environment: Setting Up Your Home and Enlisting Help

Establishing a supportive environment is essential for a successful breastfeeding journey. By setting up your home to facilitate breastfeeding and enlisting the help of supportive individuals, you can ensure that you have the resources and assistance you need to breastfeed comfortably and confidently. Here are some tips for creating a supportive environment for breastfeeding:
Designated Breastfeeding Area:

Designate a comfortable and private area in your home specifically for breastfeeding. Choose a quiet space with minimal distractions where you can relax and focus on bonding with your baby during feeding sessions.
Comfortable Seating:
Invest in a comfortable chair or nursing rocker for your breastfeeding area. Choose a chair with good back support and armrests to help you maintain proper posture during breastfeeding sessions.
Breastfeeding Supplies Within Reach:

Keep essential breastfeeding supplies, such as nursing bras, breast pads, nipple cream, and a water bottle, within easy reach of your breastfeeding area. Having these items readily available will make breastfeeding more convenient and comfortable.
Supportive Pillows:

Use supportive pillows or a nursing pillow to provide additional comfort and positioning support during breastfeeding. A well-placed pillow can help elevate your baby to the correct height and angle for a proper latch.
Breastfeeding-Friendly Clothing:

Wear breastfeeding-friendly clothing that allows for easy access during feeding sessions. Choose tops or dresses with nursing openings or front panels that can be easily lifted or unbuttoned for breastfeeding.
Enlist Supportive Partners and Family Members:

Communicate your breastfeeding goals and needs with your partner and family members, and enlist their support in creating a breastfeeding-friendly environment. Encourage them to help with household tasks and childcare responsibilities to allow you time for breastfeeding and rest.
Arrange for Professional Support:

Consider hiring a lactation consultant or attending breastfeeding support groups to receive personalized guidance and troubleshooting tips. A lactation consultant can provide valuable assistance with breastfeeding challenges and help you navigate any issues that may arise.
Educate Supportive Individuals:

Educate your partner, family members, and caregivers about the importance of breastfeeding and how they can support you in your breastfeeding journey. Provide them with information about breastfeeding techniques, positioning, and common challenges so they can offer assistance when needed.
Create a Supportive Online Community:

Join online breastfeeding support groups or forums to connect with other breastfeeding mothers and seek advice, encouragement, and camaraderie. Online communities can provide valuable peer support and reassurance during your breastfeeding journey.

By creating a supportive environment for breastfeeding and enlisting the help of supportive individuals, you can nurture a positive and empowering breastfeeding experience for both you and your baby. Remember that breastfeeding is a team effort, and having a strong support system can make all the difference in your breastfeeding success.

CHAPTER 3: THE FIRST FEW DAYS

The first few days after your baby is born are a critical time for establishing breastfeeding and bonding with your newborn. In this chapter, we will explore what to expect during this initial period, from your baby's first latch to navigating common challenges and milestones in the early days of breastfeeding.

The Golden Hour:

The first hour after birth, often referred to as the "golden hour," is an ideal time for initiating breastfeeding. Skin-to-skin contact between you and your baby during this time can promote bonding, regulate your baby's temperature and heart rate, and stimulate breastfeeding instincts.
The First Latch:

Encourage your baby to latch onto your breast as soon as possible after birth. A proper latch is essential for effective breastfeeding and milk transfer. Seek assistance from your healthcare provider or a lactation consultant if you encounter difficulties with latching.
Colostrum, the Liquid Gold:

Colostrum, often called "liquid gold," is the first milk your body produces after birth. Rich in antibodies and essential nutrients, colostrum provides valuable protection and nourishment for your newborn in the early days of life.
Frequent Feedings:

In the first few days, your baby will have small stomach capacity and frequent hunger cues. Expect to breastfeed your baby frequently, at least 8 to 12 times in a 24-hour period, to meet their nutritional needs and stimulate milk production.
Cluster Feeding:

Cluster feeding, or frequent, closely spaced feedings, is common in the early days of breastfeeding. Cluster feeding helps establish your milk supply and allows your baby to receive the colostrum-rich milk they need for optimal growth and development.
Breast Changes:

Your breasts may undergo significant changes in the first few days of breastfeeding, including engorgement, increased milk production, and changes in nipple sensitivity. Practice proper breast care, such as applying warm compresses or expressing milk to relieve engorgement and discomfort.
Seeking Support:

Don't hesitate to seek support and guidance from your healthcare provider, lactation consultant, or breastfeeding support group if you encounter challenges or have questions about breastfeeding. Early intervention and support can help address breastfeeding issues and ensure a positive breastfeeding experience for both you and your baby.
Monitoring Baby's Output:

Monitor your baby's diaper output to ensure they are receiving an adequate amount of milk. Expect your baby to have at least one wet diaper and one bowel movement on the first day of life, with increasing frequency as your milk supply increases.

Rest and Recovery:

Remember to prioritize rest and self-care in the first few days postpartum. Allow yourself time to recover from childbirth and adjust to the demands of breastfeeding. Enlist the help of supportive partners and family members to assist with household tasks and childcare responsibilities.

By understanding what to expect and seeking support when needed, you can navigate the first few days of breastfeeding with confidence and ease. Embrace this special time with your newborn, and trust in your body's ability to nourish and nurture your baby through breastfeeding.

Colostrum: Baby's First Superfood

Colostrum, often referred to as "baby's first superfood," is a miraculous substance produced by your body in the early days after childbirth. This nutrient-rich fluid is packed with antibodies, vitamins, and minerals, providing your newborn with essential nourishment and protection during their transition to the outside world. Here's why colostrum is truly nature's gift to newborns:

Rich in Antibodies: Colostrum contains a high concentration of antibodies, also known as immunoglobulins, which help protect your baby against infections and diseases. These antibodies provide passive immunity to your baby, helping to strengthen their immune system and ward off illness in the crucial early days of life.

Nutrient-Dense: Despite its small volume, colostrum is incredibly nutrient-dense, providing your baby with a concentrated source of essential nutrients, including protein, fat, vitamins, and minerals. This nutrient-rich composition supports your baby's growth, development, and overall health in the critical early stages of life.

Gentle Laxative Effect: Colostrum has a gentle laxative effect on your baby's digestive system, helping to facilitate the passage of meconium, the thick, sticky stool that accumulates in your baby's intestines during gestation. This helps clear your baby's digestive tract and prepares their body for the transition to mature milk.

Promotes Gut Health: Colostrum contains bioactive components, such as growth factors and probiotics, that promote the growth of beneficial bacteria in your baby's gut. This supports the development of a healthy microbiome, which plays a crucial role in immune function, digestion, and overall well-being.

Encourages Bonding and Attachment: Breastfeeding and skin-to-skin contact during the early days after birth promote bonding and attachment between you and your baby. The act of breastfeeding releases hormones such as oxytocin, often referred to as the "love hormone," which enhances feelings of closeness, trust, and connection between you and your baby.

Stimulates Milk Production: The frequent breastfeeding sessions in the early days after birth help stimulate your body to produce mature milk. The demand-and-supply mechanism of breastfeeding ensures that your milk supply matches your baby's evolving needs as they grow and develop.

Natural Pain Relief: Colostrum contains natural pain-relieving compounds that can soothe and comfort your baby during breastfeeding. The act of breastfeeding releases endorphins, which provide natural pain relief and promote relaxation for both you and your baby.

Emotional and Psychological Benefits: Breastfeeding and receiving colostrum provide your baby with comfort, security, and reassurance during the transition from the womb to the outside world. The close physical contact and nurturing environment of breastfeeding promote feelings of safety, warmth, and well-being for your baby.

In summary, colostrum is a true superfood for newborns, offering a wealth of benefits that support your baby's health, development, and emotional well-being in the critical early days after birth. Embrace the gift of colostrum and cherish the special bonding moments it fosters between you and your baby as you embark on your breastfeeding journey together.

Establishing Milk Supply: Ensuring a Strong Start

Establishing a robust milk supply is crucial for successful breastfeeding and ensuring that your baby receives the nourishment they need to thrive. During the early days and weeks after birth, your body undergoes a process called lactogenesis to initiate and establish milk production. Here are some essential tips for ensuring a strong start in establishing your milk supply:

Early and Frequent Nursing: Begin breastfeeding as soon as possible after birth, ideally within the first hour. Early and frequent nursing sessions stimulate your body to produce milk and help establish a healthy milk supply. Aim to breastfeed your baby at least 8 to 12 times in a 24-hour period, including night feedings.

Skin-to-Skin Contact: Practice skin-to-skin contact with your baby as much as possible, both during and between breastfeeding sessions. Skin-to-skin contact promotes bonding, regulates your baby's temperature and heart rate, and enhances milk production by stimulating the release of hormones such as oxytocin.

Emptying the Breasts: Ensure that your baby effectively empties both breasts during each feeding session. Allow your baby to nurse at the first breast until they show signs of fullness or detachment, then offer the second breast if they are still hungry. Emptying the breasts signals your body to produce more milk.

Responsive Feeding: Practice responsive feeding by breastfeeding whenever your baby shows hunger cues, such as rooting, sucking on fists, or making sucking motions. Responding promptly to your baby's hunger cues helps maintain milk production and ensures that your baby receives adequate nutrition.

Breast Compression: Use breast compression techniques during breastfeeding to maximize milk transfer and encourage your baby to nurse actively. Gentle compression of the breast can help increase milk flow and ensure that your baby receives a sufficient amount of milk during each feeding session.

Pumping and Hand Expression: If your baby is unable to breastfeed directly or if you need to supplement breastfeeding with expressed milk, consider pumping or hand expressing milk to stimulate milk production and maintain supply. Use a breast pump or hand express milk after breastfeeding sessions to empty the breasts fully.

Stay Hydrated and Nourished: Drink plenty of fluids and maintain a balanced diet rich in nutrients to support milk production and overall health. Aim to consume nutritious foods and beverages that provide essential vitamins, minerals, and hydration to support lactation.

Seek Support and Guidance: Don't hesitate to seek support and guidance from your healthcare provider, lactation consultant, or breastfeeding support group if you have concerns about milk supply or encounter challenges with breastfeeding. Professional assistance can offer reassurance, troubleshooting tips, and personalized guidance to help you establish and maintain a strong milk supply.

By implementing these strategies and prioritizing frequent nursing, responsive feeding, and supportive care, you can lay the foundation for a robust milk supply and enjoy a fulfilling breastfeeding journey with your baby. Remember that every breastfeeding journey is unique, and it's okay to seek help and support along the way as needed. Trust in your body's ability to nourish and nurture your baby through breastfeeding, and cherish the special bonding moments it brings.

Common Challenges: Troubleshooting Early Difficulties

While breastfeeding is a natural and beautiful experience, it can also present challenges for some mothers and babies in the early days. Understanding and addressing these challenges promptly can help you overcome obstacles and continue breastfeeding successfully. Here are some common breastfeeding challenges and strategies for troubleshooting them:

Latch Issues:

Challenge: Your baby may have difficulty latching onto the breast properly, leading to ineffective breastfeeding and nipple discomfort.
Solution: Seek assistance from a lactation consultant or healthcare provider to assess your baby's latch and offer guidance on proper positioning and latch techniques. Experiment with different breastfeeding positions, such as the football hold or laid-back breastfeeding, to find what works best for you and your baby.
Engorgement:

Challenge: Engorgement occurs when your breasts become swollen, firm, and painful due to an overabundance of milk.
Solution: Apply warm compresses or take a warm shower before breastfeeding to help soften the breast tissue and improve milk flow. Breastfeed frequently and ensure that your baby empties the breasts fully during each feeding session. Consider hand expressing or using a breast pump to relieve engorgement if necessary.
Sore Nipples:

Challenge: Sore nipples are a common complaint among breastfeeding mothers and can be caused by improper latch, friction, or sensitivity.
Solution: Ensure that your baby latches onto the breast correctly, with their mouth covering both the nipple and a portion of the areola. Use lanolin-based nipple cream or coconut oil to soothe and moisturize sore nipples between feedings. Experiment with different breastfeeding positions to reduce friction and pressure on tender nipples.
Low Milk Supply:

Challenge: Some mothers may experience challenges with milk production, leading to concerns about low milk supply.

Solution: Increase breastfeeding frequency by offering the breast whenever your baby shows hunger cues. Practice breast compression techniques during feeding to maximize milk transfer. Consider pumping or hand expressing milk between feedings to stimulate milk production and maintain supply. Stay hydrated and nourished, and prioritize rest and self-care to support milk production.
Latch-on Pain:

Challenge: Latch-on pain, or pain experienced when your baby first latches onto the breast, can be uncomfortable and distressing.
Solution: Address latch issues by ensuring proper positioning and latch technique. Break the latch gently if it feels uncomfortable and try again. Experiment with different breastfeeding positions to find one that minimizes discomfort. Seek assistance from a lactation consultant or healthcare provider if latch-on pain persists.
Mastitis:

Challenge: Mastitis is an inflammatory condition of the breast tissue that can cause pain, swelling, redness, and flu-like symptoms.
Solution: Rest, hydrate, and continue breastfeeding frequently to help resolve mastitis. Apply warm compresses to the affected breast and massage gently to relieve pain and promote milk flow. Seek medical attention if symptoms worsen or if you develop a fever, as antibiotics may be necessary to treat mastitis.
Tongue Tie or Lip Tie:

Challenge: Tongue tie or lip tie occurs when the tissue connecting the tongue or lip to the mouth is tight or restrictive, affecting breastfeeding latch and milk transfer.

Solution: Consult with a healthcare provider or lactation consultant to assess for tongue tie or lip tie in your baby. Depending on the severity, treatment options may include revision of the tissue through a simple procedure known as frenotomy or frenectomy.
Nipple Confusion:

Challenge: Nipple confusion occurs when a baby has difficulty transitioning between breastfeeding and bottle feeding, leading to feeding difficulties and frustration.
Solution: Minimize the use of bottles and pacifiers in the early weeks of breastfeeding to prevent nipple confusion. Practice paced bottle feeding techniques if supplementing with expressed milk to mimic the flow and pace of breastfeeding. Seek guidance from a lactation consultant if nipple confusion persists.
By recognizing and addressing these common breastfeeding challenges early on, you can overcome obstacles and continue breastfeeding successfully. Don't hesitate to seek support and guidance from your healthcare provider, lactation consultant, or breastfeeding support group if you encounter difficulties or have questions about breastfeeding. Remember that with patience, perseverance, and support, you can overcome challenges and enjoy a rewarding breastfeeding journey with your baby.

Chapter 4: Nutrition for Nursing Mothers

Proper nutrition is essential for nursing mothers to support milk production, maintain energy levels, and promote overall well-being. In this chapter, we will explore the dietary considerations and recommendations for nursing mothers to ensure optimal nutrition for both mother and baby.

Caloric Needs:

Nursing mothers have increased caloric needs to support milk production. Aim to consume an additional 300 to 500 calories per day above your pre-pregnancy intake to meet the demands of breastfeeding.

Hydration:

Staying hydrated is crucial for milk production and overall health. Drink plenty of fluids throughout the day, aiming for at least 8 to 10 cups of water or other hydrating beverages.

Balanced Diet:

Focus on consuming a balanced diet rich in fruits, vegetables, whole grains, lean proteins, and healthy fats. Include a variety of nutrient-dense foods to ensure you and your baby receive essential vitamins and minerals.

Protein-Rich Foods:

Protein is important for tissue repair and growth, making it essential for both mother and baby. Include sources of lean protein such as poultry, fish, beans, lentils, tofu, and nuts in your diet.

Healthy Fats:

Omega-3 fatty acids are beneficial for brain development and may contribute to the composition of breast milk. Incorporate sources of healthy fats such as fatty fish (salmon, mackerel, sardines), avocados, nuts, seeds, and olive oil into your meals.
Calcium-Rich Foods:

Calcium is important for bone health, both for you and your baby. Include sources of calcium such as dairy products, fortified plant-based milk alternatives, leafy greens (kale, spinach), tofu, and almonds in your diet.
Iron-Rich Foods:

Iron is essential for energy production and preventing iron deficiency anemia. Include sources of iron such as lean meats, poultry, fish, fortified cereals, beans, lentils, and dark leafy greens in your meals.
Fiber:

Fiber helps regulate digestion and prevent constipation, a common concern during the postpartum period. Include high-fiber foods such as fruits, vegetables, whole grains, beans, and legumes in your diet.
Limit Caffeine and Alcohol:

Limit your intake of caffeine and alcohol while breastfeeding, as these substances can pass into breast milk and affect your baby. Aim to consume caffeine in moderation and avoid alcohol or limit it to an occasional drink, timing it carefully around breastfeeding sessions.
Supplements:

Consider taking a prenatal vitamin or a postnatal supplement specifically formulated for breastfeeding mothers to ensure you meet your nutritional needs, particularly for vitamins D and B12, iodine, and omega-3 fatty acids.

Listen to Your Body:

Pay attention to hunger and fullness cues, and eat when you're hungry and stop when you're satisfied. Listen to your body's signals and honor your hunger and cravings while making mindful food choices.

Seek Support:

Don't hesitate to seek guidance from a registered dietitian or healthcare provider if you have questions or concerns about nutrition during breastfeeding. A professional can offer personalized recommendations and support to help you optimize your diet for breastfeeding success.

By prioritizing nutritious foods, staying hydrated, and listening to your body's cues, you can ensure that you and your baby receive the essential nutrients needed for a healthy breastfeeding journey. Remember that taking care of yourself through proper nutrition is key to providing the best start for your baby's growth and development.

Eating for Two: Nutritional Needs While Breastfeeding

Breastfeeding mothers often hear the phrase "eating for two," emphasizing the importance of adequate nutrition for both mother and baby during the lactation period. While it's true that breastfeeding requires additional energy and nutrients, it's essential to approach nutritional needs with balance and mindfulness. Here's how to nourish yourself and your baby effectively while breastfeeding:

Increased Caloric Intake:

While breastfeeding, your body requires additional calories to support milk production. However, the concept of "eating for two" doesn't mean doubling your caloric intake. Aim for an extra 300 to 500 calories per day above your pre-pregnancy intake, focusing on nutrient-dense foods that provide essential vitamins, minerals, and macronutrients.

Quality Over Quantity:

Instead of focusing solely on quantity, prioritize the quality of your calories. Choose nutrient-rich foods that offer a wide range of vitamins, minerals, antioxidants, and fiber to support your overall health and well-being. Incorporate plenty of fruits, vegetables, whole grains, lean proteins, and healthy fats into your meals and snacks.

Balanced Meals and Snacks:
Aim for balanced meals and snacks that include a combination of carbohydrates, protein, and healthy fats to provide sustained energy and satiety. Include a variety of food groups in each meal, such as whole grains, lean proteins (like chicken, fish, tofu, or beans), healthy fats (such as avocado, nuts, seeds, or olive oil), and plenty of fruits and vegetables.

Hydration:
Staying hydrated is crucial for milk production and overall health. Drink plenty of fluids throughout the day, including water, herbal teas, and other hydrating beverages. Aim to consume at least 8 to 10 cups of fluids daily, and listen to your body's thirst cues to ensure adequate hydration.

Listen to Your Body:

Pay attention to your body's hunger and fullness cues, and eat when you're hungry and stop when you're satisfied. Trust your body's wisdom to guide your food choices and portion sizes, and honor your cravings while making mindful choices that nourish both you and your baby.
Optimize Nutrient Intake:

Focus on consuming nutrient-dense foods that provide essential vitamins and minerals for both you and your baby. Prioritize foods rich in calcium, iron, omega-3 fatty acids, vitamin D, and other nutrients important for lactation and overall health.
Meal Timing and Frequency:

Eat regular, balanced meals and snacks throughout the day to maintain stable blood sugar levels and support energy levels and milk production. Aim to eat every 3 to 4 hours, including a combination of meals and snacks to keep hunger at bay and prevent energy dips.
Supplements:

In addition to a balanced diet, consider taking a prenatal vitamin or a postnatal supplement specifically formulated for breastfeeding mothers to ensure you meet your nutritional needs. Talk to your healthcare provider about supplement recommendations tailored to your individual needs. Remember that every breastfeeding journey is unique, and your nutritional needs may vary based on factors such as age, weight, activity level, and overall health. Listen to your body, prioritize self-care, and seek support from healthcare providers, lactation consultants, and other breastfeeding support resources as needed to ensure a healthy and fulfilling breastfeeding experience for both you and your baby.

Hydration and Milk Supply: Importance of Staying Hydrated

Staying hydrated is crucial for breastfeeding mothers, as adequate hydration plays a significant role in milk production and overall lactation success. Here's why staying hydrated is essential for maintaining a healthy milk supply:

Optimal Milk Production:

Breast milk is composed of approximately 88% water, making hydration essential for producing an ample milk supply. When you're adequately hydrated, your body can efficiently produce and release milk to meet your baby's feeding needs. Regulating Body Fluids:

Hydration helps regulate your body's fluid balance, ensuring that you maintain adequate blood volume and hydration levels throughout the day. Proper fluid balance supports overall bodily functions, including milk production and secretion.
Preventing Dehydration:

Dehydration can negatively impact milk production and quality, leading to a decrease in milk supply and potential feeding difficulties for your baby. By staying hydrated, you can prevent dehydration and maintain optimal milk flow and volume.
Supporting Baby's Hydration:

Adequate hydration for the breastfeeding mother ensures that your baby receives well-hydrated breast milk, which is essential for their hydration and overall health. Breast milk provides the perfect balance of water and nutrients to keep your baby hydrated and satisfied.
Boosting Energy Levels:

Hydration supports energy levels and overall well-being, helping you feel more alert, focused, and energized throughout the day. By staying hydrated, you can better cope with the demands of breastfeeding and caring for your baby. Optimizing Postpartum Recovery:

Proper hydration is crucial for postpartum recovery, helping your body heal and replenish fluids lost during childbirth. By prioritizing hydration, you can support your body's recovery process and promote overall health and well-being. Preventing Common Concerns:

Adequate hydration can help prevent common breastfeeding concerns such as engorgement, plugged ducts, and mastitis. By staying hydrated, you can maintain optimal breast health and reduce the risk of complications associated with breastfeeding.
To ensure adequate hydration while breastfeeding, aim to drink plenty of fluids throughout the day, including water, herbal teas, and other hydrating beverages. Pay attention to your body's thirst cues and drink fluids whenever you feel thirsty, as well as during breastfeeding sessions and throughout the day. Additionally, limit your intake of caffeinated and alcoholic beverages, as these can have diuretic effects and contribute to dehydration.

By prioritizing hydration and staying mindful of your fluid intake, you can support optimal milk production, maintain your energy levels, and promote overall health and well-being for both you and your baby during the breastfeeding journey.

Foods to Avoid: What to Steer Clear of During Breastfeeding

While breastfeeding, it's important to be mindful of your dietary choices to ensure that you and your baby remain healthy and comfortable. While most foods are safe to consume while breastfeeding, some may cause discomfort or adverse reactions in breastfeeding infants. Here are some foods to consider avoiding or consuming in moderation while breastfeeding:

Caffeine:

While moderate caffeine intake is generally considered safe for breastfeeding mothers, excessive caffeine consumption can lead to irritability, restlessness, and sleep disturbances in breastfeeding infants. Limit your intake of caffeinated beverages such as coffee, tea, and soda, and be mindful of caffeine content in medications and supplements.
Alcohol:

Alcohol can pass into breast milk and affect your baby's sleep patterns, behavior, and development. Avoid excessive alcohol consumption while breastfeeding, and if you choose to drink alcohol, limit it to an occasional drink and time it carefully around breastfeeding sessions to minimize exposure to your baby.
Fish High in Mercury:

Certain types of fish, particularly large predatory fish such as shark, swordfish, king mackerel, and tilefish, may contain high levels of mercury, which can be harmful to your baby's developing nervous system. Limit consumption of these fish and opt for varieties lower in mercury, such as salmon, trout, sardines, and anchovies.
Allergenic Foods:

Some breastfeeding infants may be sensitive or allergic to certain foods commonly associated with allergies, such as cow's milk, eggs, peanuts, tree nuts, soy, wheat, fish, and shellfish. If you have a family history of food allergies or notice signs of allergic reactions in your baby, consider eliminating potential allergens from your diet and consult with a healthcare provider or allergist for guidance.
Spicy Foods:

Spicy foods can sometimes cause gastrointestinal discomfort or irritation in breastfeeding infants, leading to fussiness or digestive issues. While occasional consumption of spicy foods is unlikely to cause harm, be mindful of your baby's reactions and adjust your diet accordingly if necessary.
Gas-Producing Foods:

Some foods known to produce gas, such as beans, broccoli, cabbage, onions, and garlic, may cause discomfort or increased gas in breastfeeding infants. While these foods are nutritious and beneficial for breastfeeding mothers, consider consuming them in moderation and observing your baby's reactions.
Strong Flavors and Odors:

Foods with strong flavors or odors, such as garlic, onions, and certain spices, may affect the taste and smell of breast milk, potentially influencing your baby's acceptance of breastfeeding. While these foods are generally safe to consume, be mindful of your baby's preferences and reactions.
Artificial Sweeteners:

Some artificial sweeteners, such as saccharin and aspartame, may pass into breast milk in small amounts and could potentially affect your baby. While most artificial sweeteners are considered safe for breastfeeding mothers when consumed in moderation, consider limiting your intake or opting for natural sweeteners such as stevia or honey.

Remember that every breastfeeding mother and baby is unique, and what works well for one may not be the same for another. Pay attention to your baby's reactions to different foods and make adjustments to your diet as needed to ensure a comfortable and healthy breastfeeding experience for both you and your baby. If you have specific concerns or questions about your diet while breastfeeding, consult with a healthcare provider or registered dietitian for personalized guidance and recommendations.

Breastfeeding is a natural and beautiful experience, but it can also come with its share of challenges. In this chapter, we will explore some of the common breastfeeding issues that mothers may encounter and provide practical tips and strategies for overcoming them.

Engorgement:

Engorgement occurs when the breasts become overly full of milk, leading to discomfort and difficulty latching. To alleviate engorgement, try applying warm compresses or taking a warm shower before nursing to encourage milk flow. Massaging the breasts and expressing a small amount of milk by hand or with a breast pump can also help relieve pressure and facilitate easier latching for your baby.
Sore Nipples:

Sore nipples are a common concern for breastfeeding mothers, especially in the early days. Ensure that your baby is latching correctly to minimize nipple pain, and consider using lanolin cream or nipple shields to soothe soreness between feedings. Alternating breastfeeding positions and allowing your nipples to air dry after nursing can also promote healing and reduce discomfort.
Low Milk Supply:

Low milk supply can be stressful for breastfeeding mothers, but there are several strategies you can try to increase milk production. Ensure frequent and effective breastfeeding or pumping sessions to stimulate milk production, and consider using breast compression techniques during nursing to encourage milk flow. Adequate hydration, nutrition, and rest are also essential for maintaining a healthy milk supply, so prioritize self-care and seek support from a lactation consultant or healthcare provider if needed.
Latch Issues:

A proper latch is crucial for effective breastfeeding and preventing nipple pain and damage. If you're experiencing latch issues, seek guidance from a lactation consultant or breastfeeding specialist who can assess your baby's latch and provide personalized recommendations for improvement. Experimenting with different breastfeeding positions, ensuring proper positioning and support for both you and your baby, and offering gentle guidance to encourage a deeper latch can also help resolve latch problems.
Mastitis:

Mastitis is an inflammation of the breast tissue that can cause pain, swelling, redness, and flu-like symptoms. To relieve mastitis symptoms, rest as much as possible, apply warm compresses to the affected breast, and continue breastfeeding or pumping frequently to maintain milk flow and prevent further congestion. If symptoms persist or worsen, seek medical attention promptly for antibiotic treatment and support.

Blocked Milk Ducts:

Blocked milk ducts occur when milk flow becomes obstructed, leading to localized pain, swelling, and tenderness in the breast. To clear blocked ducts, apply warm compresses and gently massage the affected area while breastfeeding or pumping. Ensure proper breast drainage by alternating breastfeeding positions and using gravity-assisted techniques such as leaning forward while nursing. Continued breastfeeding or pumping is essential to prevent further blockage and promote healing.
Thrush:

Thrush is a fungal infection caused by Candida yeast that can affect the nipples and breast tissue, causing pain, itching, and white patches in the baby's mouth. Treatment typically involves antifungal medication for both mother and baby, as well as practicing good hygiene and sterilizing breastfeeding equipment to prevent reinfection. If you suspect thrush, consult with a healthcare provider for diagnosis and treatment options.
Breastfeeding in Public:

Breastfeeding in public can feel daunting for some mothers, but with practice and confidence, it can become a comfortable and empowering experience. Familiarize yourself with your legal rights regarding breastfeeding in public, and consider using nursing-friendly clothing or accessories to discreetly nurse your baby while out and about. Remember that breastfeeding is a natural and beautiful act, and you have the right to feed your baby wherever you feel comfortable and supported.

By addressing common breastfeeding issues proactively and seeking support when needed, you can overcome challenges and enjoy a fulfilling breastfeeding journey with your baby. Remember that every breastfeeding experience is unique, and it's okay to ask for help and support along the way. Trust your instincts as a mother and prioritize your well-being and that of your baby as you navigate the joys and challenges of breastfeeding.

Latching Problems: Tips for Improving Latch

A proper latch is essential for successful breastfeeding, as it ensures efficient milk transfer and prevents nipple pain and damage. If you're experiencing latching problems with your baby, here are some tips to help improve latch and enhance your breastfeeding experience:

Positioning:

Experiment with different breastfeeding positions to find one that works best for you and your baby. Common positions include the cradle hold, football hold, side-lying position, and laid-back breastfeeding. Choose a position that allows your baby to approach the breast with their mouth wide open and chin touching the breast first.
Nose to Nipple:

When latching your baby, aim to bring their nose to the level of your nipple, with their mouth wide open. This allows for a deeper latch and better milk flow. Gently tickle your baby's upper lip with your nipple to encourage them to open their mouth wide before latching.
Support:

Provide adequate support for your breast and your baby during breastfeeding. Use your hand to shape your breast into a "sandwich" or "C" shape, with your fingers positioned away from the areola to allow your baby to latch deeply. Support your baby's neck and shoulders with your hand or arm, ensuring that they are positioned close to you and facing your breast.
Wait for the Wide Mouth:

Wait for your baby to open their mouth wide before bringing them to the breast. This allows for a deeper latch and better positioning of the nipple in your baby's mouth. Look for signs of hunger such as rooting, sucking motions, and hand-to-mouth movements before offering the breast.
Chin First:

Encourage your baby to latch onto the breast chin first, with their lower lip flanged outwards and their tongue extended over the lower gumline. This helps ensure that your baby takes in a good mouthful of breast tissue, rather than just the nipple, reducing the risk of nipple pain and damage.
Break the Seal:

If your baby is having difficulty latching deeply, gently break the suction by inserting your finger into the corner of their mouth and pressing down on their chin to release the latch. Then, reposition your baby and try latching again, ensuring that they achieve a deeper latch.
Seek Support:

If you're struggling with latching issues, don't hesitate to seek support from a lactation consultant, breastfeeding counselor, or healthcare provider. They can assess your baby's latch, provide personalized guidance and support, and help you troubleshoot any challenges you may be facing.
Patience and Persistence:

Remember that learning to breastfeed takes time and practice for both you and your baby. Be patient with yourself and your baby as you work together to improve latch and establish a comfortable breastfeeding routine. Celebrate small victories along the way and seek support from your partner, family, and friends as needed.

By incorporating these tips into your breastfeeding routine and seeking support when needed, you can improve latch and enjoy a positive breastfeeding experience with your baby. Trust in your body's ability to breastfeed and nurture your baby, and remember that each feeding session is an opportunity to bond and connect with your little one.

Sore Nipples and Breast Pain: Prevention and Treatment

Sore nipples and breast pain are common concerns for breastfeeding mothers, especially in the early days of breastfeeding. Fortunately, there are steps you can take to prevent and alleviate soreness and discomfort, ensuring a more comfortable breastfeeding experience for you and your baby. Here are some tips for prevention and treatment:

Prevention:

Proper Latch:

Ensure that your baby is latching correctly to the breast, with their mouth wide open and taking in a good mouthful of breast tissue. A deep latch helps distribute the pressure evenly on the nipple and areola, reducing the risk of soreness and damage.

Positioning:

Experiment with different breastfeeding positions to find one that is comfortable and effective for you and your baby. Avoid positions that put unnecessary strain on your nipples or breast tissue.
Break the Seal Gently:

If your baby has difficulty latching deeply or you feel discomfort during breastfeeding, gently break the suction by inserting your finger into the corner of their mouth and pressing down on their chin to release the latch. Then, reposition your baby and try latching again.
Air Dry:
After breastfeeding, allow your nipples to air dry before covering them with clothing or breast pads. Moisture trapped against the skin can contribute to nipple soreness and irritation.
Avoid Harsh Soaps:

Avoid using harsh soaps or lotions on your nipples, as these can strip away natural oils and cause dryness and irritation. Stick to mild, unscented cleansers when washing your breasts.
Treatment:

Lanolin Cream:

Apply lanolin cream or nipple balm to your nipples after breastfeeding to soothe soreness and promote healing. Lanolin is safe for breastfeeding and provides a protective barrier against further irritation.
Warm Compresses:

Apply warm compresses to your breasts before breastfeeding to help soften the breast tissue and alleviate discomfort. You can also use warm compresses between feedings to relieve soreness and promote relaxation.

Cool Compresses:
After breastfeeding, apply cool compresses or chilled cabbage leaves to your breasts to reduce swelling and inflammation. The cool temperature can help numb the area and provide relief from soreness.
Breast Shields:
Consider using soft breast shields or silicone nipple protectors between feedings to protect your nipples from friction and irritation. Breast shields can also help promote healing by allowing air to circulate around the nipple.
Pain Relievers:

Over-the-counter pain relievers such as ibuprofen or acetaminophen can help alleviate breast pain and discomfort. Always consult with a healthcare provider before taking any medication while breastfeeding.
Rest and Relaxation:

Prioritize rest and relaxation to allow your body time to heal. Take breaks throughout the day to rest and bond with your baby, and enlist the help of your partner, family, or friends with household chores and childcare responsibilities.
Seek Support:

If you're experiencing persistent nipple soreness or breast pain, seek support from a lactation consultant, breastfeeding counselor, or healthcare provider. They can assess your breastfeeding technique, provide personalized recommendations, and help you address any underlying issues contributing to your discomfort.

By taking proactive steps to prevent and treat sore nipples and breast pain, you can promote a more comfortable and enjoyable breastfeeding experience for both you and your baby. Remember that it's normal to experience some discomfort in the early days of breastfeeding, but persistent pain or soreness may indicate a need for further evaluation and support. Trust your instincts as a mother and reach out for help when needed, knowing that support is available to help you navigate the challenges of breastfeeding with confidence and ease.

Low Milk Supply: Strategies to Boost Production

Low milk supply can be a source of stress and concern for breastfeeding mothers, but there are several strategies you can try to increase milk production and ensure an ample milk supply for your baby. Here are some effective strategies to boost milk production:

Frequent Nursing or Pumping:

Breastfeeding works on the principle of supply and demand, so the more often you breastfeed or pump, the more milk your body will produce. Aim to breastfeed your baby on demand, offering the breast whenever they show signs of hunger, and consider adding additional pumping sessions between feedings to stimulate milk production further.
Effective Milk Removal:

Ensure that your baby is effectively removing milk from the breast during breastfeeding or pumping sessions. A poor latch or inefficient milk transfer can contribute to low milk supply. Work with a lactation consultant or breastfeeding specialist to assess your baby's latch and feeding technique and make any necessary adjustments to improve milk removal.
Skin-to-Skin Contact:

Practice skin-to-skin contact with your baby as much as possible, especially in the early days and weeks after birth. Skin-to-skin contact stimulates the release of oxytocin, the hormone responsible for milk ejection, and promotes bonding between you and your baby. Spend time cuddling, holding, and nursing your baby skin-to-skin to enhance milk production and breastfeeding success.
Galactagogues:

Galactagogues are substances that are believed to increase milk supply. Common galactagogues include oatmeal, fenugreek, blessed thistle, and brewer's yeast. Incorporate these foods into your diet or consider taking herbal supplements under the guidance of a healthcare provider to support milk production. Be cautious when using herbal supplements and discontinue use if you experience any adverse effects.
Hydration and Nutrition:

Stay well-hydrated and consume a balanced diet rich in nutrients to support milk production. Drink plenty of water throughout the day, and eat a variety of foods that are high in protein, healthy fats, vitamins, and minerals. Foods such as whole grains, lean proteins, fruits, vegetables, and dairy products can help nourish your body and support optimal milk production.
Breast Compression:

During breastfeeding or pumping sessions, practice breast compression techniques to help empty the breast more effectively and stimulate milk production. Use your hand to gently compress and massage the breast while your baby is nursing or while you're pumping to encourage milk flow and drainage.
Rest and Relaxation:

Prioritize rest and relaxation to support milk production and overall well-being. Take breaks throughout the day to rest, nap, or engage in activities that help you relax and unwind. Stress and fatigue can negatively impact milk supply, so it's essential to prioritize self-care and seek support from your partner, family, and friends as needed.

Seek Support:

If you're struggling with low milk supply despite trying these strategies, seek support from a lactation consultant, breastfeeding counselor, or healthcare provider. They can assess your breastfeeding technique, offer personalized guidance and support, and help you address any underlying issues contributing to low milk supply, such as tongue tie, hormonal imbalances, or medical conditions.

By implementing these strategies and seeking support when needed, you can boost milk production and ensure a plentiful milk supply for your baby's nutritional needs. Remember that every breastfeeding journey is unique, and it's okay to ask for help and support along the way. Trust your body's ability to nourish and nurture your baby, and celebrate each breastfeeding success as you bond with your little one.

CHAPTER 6: BREASTFEEDING TECHNIQUES AND TIPS

Breastfeeding is a natural and beautiful way to nourish and bond with your baby, but it can also come with its challenges. In this chapter, we will explore various breastfeeding techniques and provide tips to help you overcome common hurdles and make breastfeeding a more comfortable and enjoyable experience for both you and your baby.
Correct Latching Technique:

A proper latch is crucial for successful breastfeeding. To ensure a good latch, position your baby so that their mouth is wide open and their lips are flanged outwards, covering a large portion of the areola. Aim to bring your baby to the breast rather than leaning over to them, and support their neck and shoulders to help them maintain a comfortable position.
Engorgement Relief:

Engorgement, or the overfull feeling of the breasts, can occur in the early days of breastfeeding as your milk supply adjusts to your baby's needs. To relieve engorgement, apply warm compresses to your breasts before nursing to help soften the breast tissue and encourage milk flow. Breastfeed frequently to drain the breasts and relieve pressure, and gently massage your breasts while nursing to encourage milk flow.
Breast Compression:

Breast compression is a technique used to help your baby get more milk during breastfeeding. To perform breast compression, gently squeeze and compress your breast while your baby is nursing, mimicking the action of a milk duct and encouraging milk flow. This technique can be especially helpful for babies who have difficulty effectively removing milk from the breast or for mothers with low milk supply.
Switch Nursing:

Switch nursing involves switching back and forth between breasts during a feeding session to ensure that your baby gets enough milk from both breasts. This technique can help stimulate milk production and prevent engorgement in one breast while ensuring that your baby receives adequate nutrition. Pay attention to your baby's feeding cues and switch breasts when they show signs of slowing down or becoming disinterested.
Breastfeeding Positions:
Experiment with different breastfeeding positions to find one that is comfortable and effective for you and your baby. Common breastfeeding positions include the cradle hold, football hold, cross-cradle hold, and side-lying position. Choose a position that allows your baby to latch deeply and nurse effectively while also being comfortable for you.
Burping Techniques:

Burping your baby during and after breastfeeding can help prevent gas and discomfort. To burp your baby, hold them upright against your chest or over your shoulder and gently pat or rub their back until they release any trapped air. Burp your baby periodically during feeding sessions, especially if they seem fussy or gassy.
Cluster Feeding:

Cluster feeding, or feeding your baby more frequently for short periods of time, is common during growth spurts or developmental milestones. Cluster feeding helps boost milk supply and ensures that your baby gets enough nutrition during times of increased demand. Be patient and responsive to your baby's feeding cues during cluster feeding periods, and offer comfort and reassurance as needed.
Seeking Support:

If you're struggling with breastfeeding or have questions or concerns, don't hesitate to seek support from a lactation consultant, breastfeeding counselor, or healthcare provider. They can assess your breastfeeding technique, offer personalized guidance and support, and help you address any challenges or issues you may be experiencing.
By incorporating these breastfeeding techniques and tips into your breastfeeding routine, you can overcome common challenges and enjoy a more comfortable and fulfilling breastfeeding experience with your baby. Remember to be patient and gentle with yourself and your baby as you navigate the ups and downs of breastfeeding, and don't hesitate to reach out for support when needed.

Hand Expression: Learning the Basics

Hand expression is a valuable skill that allows you to express breast milk manually without the need for a breast pump. Whether you're looking to relieve engorgement, stimulate milk production, or collect milk for storage, mastering hand expression can be a useful tool in your breastfeeding toolkit. Here are the basics of hand expression:

Wash Your Hands:

Before you begin hand expression, wash your hands thoroughly with soap and warm water to ensure cleanliness and minimize the risk of contamination.
Find a Comfortable Position:

Sit in a comfortable chair with good back support, or lie down on your side if preferred. Make sure you're relaxed and free from distractions to facilitate milk let-down.
Massage Your Breasts:

Gently massage your breasts using circular motions, starting from the outer areas and working your way towards the nipple. This can help stimulate milk flow and make hand expression more effective.
Place Your Fingers:

Cup your breast with one hand, placing your thumb above the areola and your fingers below, forming a "C" shape around the breast. Avoid placing your fingers too close to the nipple to prevent discomfort.
Apply Pressure:

Apply gentle pressure towards the chest wall, compressing the milk ducts and encouraging milk to flow towards the nipple. Experiment with different amounts of pressure and hand movements to find what works best for you.
Express Milk:

Begin expressing milk by pressing your thumb and fingers together in a rolling motion towards the nipple. Continue to compress and release, moving your fingers around the breast to express milk from different areas.
Capture Milk:

Position a clean container or breast milk storage bag beneath your breast to capture the expressed milk. Alternatively, you can express milk directly into a clean cup or bowl if immediate feeding is anticipated.
Switch Sides:

Once you've expressed milk from one breast, switch to the other breast and repeat the process. Aim to express milk from both breasts evenly to maintain milk supply and prevent engorgement.
Practice Patience:

Hand expression may take some time and practice to master, so be patient with yourself as you learn this skill. Relax, take deep breaths, and focus on the sensations in your breasts to facilitate milk let-down.
Store Expressed Milk:

If you're collecting milk for storage, label the container with the date and time of expression and store it in the refrigerator or freezer according to recommended guidelines for safe breast milk storage.
Hand expression is a gentle and effective way to express breast milk when a breast pump is not available or practical. With practice and patience, you can become proficient in hand expression and harness its benefits to support your breastfeeding journey. If you encounter any difficulties or have questions about hand expression, don't hesitate to seek guidance from a lactation consultant or breastfeeding support professional.

Pumping Essentials: Choosing and Using a Breast Pump

Breast pumps are valuable tools that allow breastfeeding mothers to express milk and maintain their milk supply, especially when separated from their babies or when faced with breastfeeding challenges. Choosing the right breast pump and understanding how to use it effectively can make a significant difference in your breastfeeding journey. Here's what you need to know about pumping essentials:

Types of Breast Pumps:

There are three main types of breast pumps: manual, electric, and hospital-grade.
Manual pumps are operated by hand and are lightweight, portable, and quiet, making them ideal for occasional use or when on the go.
Electric pumps are powered by electricity or batteries and offer adjustable suction levels and pumping patterns for efficient milk expression. They are suitable for frequent or long-term use and come in single and double pump models.
Hospital-grade pumps are high-powered electric pumps designed for heavy-duty use and are often recommended for mothers who need to establish or maintain their milk supply, premature infants, or mothers of multiples.
Choosing the Right Pump:

Consider your breastfeeding goals, lifestyle, and pumping needs when selecting a breast pump. If you plan to pump occasionally, a manual or single electric pump may suffice. For frequent or long-term pumping, a double electric pump offers efficiency and convenience. Hospital-grade pumps are typically available for rental and may be recommended in specific situations by a healthcare provider or lactation consultant.
Getting Started:

Familiarize yourself with your breast pump by reading the instruction manual and watching instructional videos provided by the manufacturer. Assemble the pump according to the manufacturer's guidelines and ensure all components are clean and sterile before use.

Choosing the Right Flange Size:

The flange, or breast shield, is the part of the breast pump that fits over your nipple and areola. It's essential to choose the correct flange size to ensure optimal comfort and efficiency during pumping. Most breast pump manufacturers offer a range of flange sizes to accommodate different breast shapes and sizes. Experiment with different flange sizes to find the one that fits you best and allows for maximum milk flow.

Establishing a Pumping Routine:

Establish a regular pumping routine based on your baby's feeding schedule and your personal preferences. Aim to pump at least every 2-3 hours, or whenever your baby would typically nurse, to maintain your milk supply and meet your baby's nutritional needs. Use a timer or breastfeeding app to track your pumping sessions and ensure consistency.

Proper Pumping Technique:

When pumping, position the breast pump flanges over your breasts, ensuring a secure seal around your nipple and areola. Start with a low suction level and gradually increase to a comfortable level that mimics your baby's nursing pattern. Massage your breasts before and during pumping to encourage milk let-down, and relax and visualize your baby to promote milk flow.

Storing Expressed Milk:

Store expressed breast milk in clean, sterilized containers or breast milk storage bags labeled with the date and time of expression. Follow recommended guidelines for safe breast milk storage, including refrigeration or freezing as needed. Use expressed milk within the recommended storage timeframe to ensure its freshness and nutritional quality.

Cleaning and Maintenance:

After each pumping session, disassemble the breast pump and wash all parts that come into contact with breast milk with warm, soapy water. Rinse thoroughly and allow the parts to air dry or sanitize them according to the manufacturer's instructions. Regularly inspect your breast pump for signs of wear or damage and replace any worn or malfunctioning parts promptly.

By choosing the right breast pump, establishing a pumping routine, and using proper pumping technique, you can effectively express breast milk and maintain your milk supply to support your breastfeeding goals. If you have any questions or concerns about pumping or breastfeeding, don't hesitate to seek guidance from a lactation consultant or breastfeeding support professional.

Combining Breast and Bottle: Introducing the Bottle Without Weaning

Introducing the bottle while continuing to breastfeed can offer flexibility and convenience for breastfeeding mothers, allowing them to share feeding responsibilities with partners or caregivers and maintain their milk supply. However, transitioning between breast and bottle feeding requires careful consideration and patience to ensure a smooth and successful experience for both you and your baby. Here are some tips for combining breast and bottle feeding without weaning:

Timing is Key:

Introduce the bottle gradually when your baby is around 4-6 weeks old or whenever breastfeeding is well-established. Starting too early may cause nipple confusion or preference for the bottle, while waiting too long may make it more challenging for your baby to accept the bottle.
Choose the Right Bottle and Nipple:

Select a bottle and nipple that closely mimic the shape, size, and flow of the breast to help prevent nipple confusion and encourage your baby to latch onto the bottle. Look for slow-flow or newborn nipples to match the slower flow of breast milk and reduce the risk of overfeeding.
Practice Pace Feeding:

Practice paced bottle feeding techniques to mimic the natural rhythm and pace of breastfeeding. Hold the bottle horizontally, allowing the milk to flow slowly, and pause frequently to give your baby a chance to swallow and rest. This helps prevent overfeeding, reduces the risk of gas or reflux, and encourages your baby to eat more slowly and mindfully.
Offer the Bottle at the Right Time:

Offer the bottle when your baby is calm and alert but not overly hungry or tired. Avoid waiting until your baby is extremely hungry or fussy, as they may become frustrated and resistant to trying something new. Experiment with different times of day and feeding cues to find the most opportune moments for bottle feeding.

Use Breast Milk for Bottle Feeding:

Whenever possible, offer expressed breast milk in the bottle to provide the same nutritional benefits as breastfeeding and maintain your milk supply. Express milk using a breast pump or hand expression and store it in clean, sterilized containers or breast milk storage bags labeled with the date and time of expression.

Stay Involved During Bottle Feeding:

Remain actively involved during bottle feeding sessions to maintain your bond with your baby and monitor their feeding cues and behaviors. Hold your baby close, make eye contact, and talk or sing to them to promote bonding and interaction during feeding.

Be Patient and Persistent:

It may take time for your baby to adjust to bottle feeding, especially if they're accustomed to breastfeeding. Be patient and persistent, offering the bottle regularly and providing gentle encouragement and reassurance. Offer praise and positive reinforcement when your baby accepts the bottle and successfully feeds from it.

Monitor Feeding Progress:

Pay attention to your baby's feeding cues and behaviors to gauge their comfort and satisfaction during bottle feeding. Look for signs of hunger or fullness, such as rooting, sucking, swallowing, or turning away from the bottle. Adjust the feeding pace, position, or bottle nipple as needed to ensure a comfortable and enjoyable feeding experience for your baby.

By following these tips and being patient and responsive to your baby's needs, you can successfully introduce the bottle without weaning and maintain your breastfeeding relationship while offering flexibility and convenience for both you and your baby. If you encounter any challenges or concerns during the transition to bottle feeding, don't hesitate to seek guidance from a lactation consultant or breastfeeding support professional.

Chapter 7: Breastfeeding and Working

Balancing breastfeeding with a return to work can present unique challenges for mothers, but with careful planning and support, it's entirely possible to continue breastfeeding while pursuing your career goals. In this chapter, we'll explore strategies for successfully combining breastfeeding and working, ensuring that you can provide the best possible nutrition for your baby while thriving professionally.

Understanding Your Rights:

Familiarize yourself with the laws and regulations in your country or region regarding breastfeeding and employment. Many countries have laws that protect a mother's right to breastfeed or express milk in the workplace, including provisions for break time and private space for pumping.

Communicating with Your Employer:

Initiate a conversation with your employer before returning to work to discuss your plans for breastfeeding or expressing milk. Clearly communicate your needs and concerns, and work together to develop a plan that accommodates your breastfeeding schedule while meeting the demands of your job.

Creating a Pumping Schedule:

Establish a pumping schedule that aligns with your work hours and allows you to maintain your milk supply. Aim to pump at least every 3-4 hours, or as frequently as your baby would typically nurse, to prevent engorgement and ensure an adequate milk supply.

Setting Up a Pumping Space:

Advocate for a designated pumping space in your workplace that provides privacy, comfort, and access to electrical outlets. Ideally, this space should be clean, quiet, and equipped with a comfortable chair and a table or countertop for your pump and accessories.

Storing Expressed Milk:

Invest in a high-quality breast pump and storage containers or breast milk storage bags for safely expressing, storing, and transporting your breast milk. Label each container with the date and time of expression and follow recommended guidelines for safe breast milk storage and handling.

Maximizing Efficiency:

Streamline your pumping sessions to maximize efficiency and minimize disruption to your workday. Consider using hands-free pumping bras or pumping attachments that allow you to multitask while expressing milk, such as checking emails or making phone calls.

Maintaining Work-Life Balance:

Prioritize self-care and work-life balance to prevent burnout and maintain your physical and emotional well-being. Take regular breaks throughout the day to rest, eat nutritious meals, and stay hydrated, and delegate tasks or seek support from colleagues when needed.

Seeking Support:

Surround yourself with a supportive network of family, friends, and colleagues who understand and respect your breastfeeding goals. Join online communities or support groups for breastfeeding mothers in similar situations to share experiences, advice, and encouragement.

Flexibility and Adaptability:

Be prepared to adapt and adjust your breastfeeding and pumping routine as your work responsibilities and schedule evolve. Stay flexible and open-minded, and don't hesitate to revisit your pumping plan or seek assistance if challenges arise.

By implementing these strategies and advocating for your needs as a breastfeeding working mother, you can successfully navigate the transition back to work while continuing to provide the best possible nutrition for your baby through breastfeeding. Remember that every mother's journey is unique, so trust your instincts and do what works best for you and your family.

Planning for Return to Work: How to Prepare

Returning to work after maternity leave can be both exciting and daunting, especially when you're breastfeeding. However, with careful planning and preparation, you can navigate this transition smoothly and continue providing breast milk for your baby. Here are some steps to help you prepare for your return to work while maintaining your breastfeeding goals:

Know Your Rights:

Familiarize yourself with your workplace's policies and your legal rights regarding breastfeeding and pumping at work. Understand your entitlement to breaks and a private space for expressing milk, as well as any accommodations or support available to breastfeeding employees.

Start Pumping Early:

Begin pumping and storing breast milk a few weeks before you return to work to build up a stash and get your baby accustomed to taking a bottle. Start with one pumping session per day, preferably in the morning when milk supply is typically highest, to gradually increase your milk reserves.
Establish a Pumping Routine:

Plan out your pumping schedule for when you're at work based on your baby's feeding patterns and your work hours. Aim to pump every 3-4 hours, or as frequently as your baby would typically nurse, to maintain your milk supply and prevent engorgement.
Set Up a Pumping Station:

Create a dedicated pumping area at work that's comfortable, private, and equipped with a power outlet. Advocate for a clean and quiet space where you can relax and express milk without interruptions. Consider bringing your own pumping supplies, such as a pump, storage containers, and cleaning supplies, to ensure hygiene and convenience.
Communicate with Your Employer:

Have a candid conversation with your employer or HR department about your plans for breastfeeding and pumping at work. Discuss your pumping needs, schedule, and any accommodations you may require, such as flexible break times or access to a refrigerator for storing expressed milk.
Prepare Your Breastfeeding Supplies:
Pack a breastfeeding kit with all the essentials you'll need for pumping at work, including your breast pump, storage bags or bottles, spare parts, nursing pads, and comfortable clothing. Consider investing in a hands-free pumping bra or pumping accessories to make pumping sessions more efficient.
Plan Your Childcare Arrangements:

Research and secure childcare arrangements that align with your breastfeeding goals and preferences. Communicate your breastfeeding schedule and milk storage guidelines to your childcare provider, and ensure they're equipped to handle and store expressed breast milk safely.
Practice Self-Care:

Prioritize self-care and stress management as you prepare for your return to work. Get plenty of rest, eat nutritious meals, and engage in activities that help you relax and recharge. Reach out to your support network for emotional support and practical assistance as needed.
Stay Flexible and Patient:

Be prepared for unexpected challenges or adjustments as you navigate the transition back to work. Stay flexible and patient with yourself as you establish a new routine, and don't hesitate to seek help or advice from lactation consultants, breastfeeding support groups, or fellow working mothers.
By taking proactive steps to plan and prepare for your return to work while breastfeeding, you can set yourself up for success and continue providing the best possible nutrition for your baby. Remember that every breastfeeding journey is unique, so trust your instincts and be kind to yourself as you navigate this exciting new chapter.

Pumping at Work: Creating a Schedule and Finding a Private Space Pumping breast milk at work is essential for many breastfeeding mothers who are returning to their jobs. Establishing a pumping schedule and finding a private space to express milk are crucial aspects of successfully combining breastfeeding with your professional responsibilities. Here's how to create a pumping schedule and secure a private space at work:

Create a Pumping Schedule:

Plan your pumping sessions around your work schedule and
your baby's feeding routine. Aim to pump every 3-4 hours, or
as often as your baby would typically nurse, to maintain your
milk supply and prevent engorgement. Coordinate your
pumping breaks with your regular work breaks or lunch hour
whenever possible.
Communicate with Your Employer:

Notify your employer or HR department about your intention
to pump breast milk at work well in advance of your return
date. Discuss your pumping schedule and any
accommodations you may need, such as flexible break times
or a designated pumping area. Be clear about your rights as a
breastfeeding employee and advocate for the support you
require.
Identify a Pumping Location:

Scout out potential pumping locations in your workplace,
such as a designated lactation room, a private office, or a clean
and quiet area. Look for a space that provides privacy,
comfort, and access to electrical outlets for your breast pump.
Consider factors like proximity to your workspace,
convenience, and availability throughout the day.
Request Accommodations:

If your workplace doesn't already have a designated lactation
room, advocate for the creation of one or request alternative
accommodations for pumping. Present your employer with
specific suggestions for suitable pumping spaces and any
necessary modifications, such as installing a lock on the door
or adding comfortable seating.
Set Up Your Pumping Station:

Once you've identified a pumping location, set up your pumping station with all the necessary equipment and supplies. Bring your breast pump, storage bags or bottles, cleaning supplies, and any personal items you may need for comfort. Consider investing in a hands-free pumping bra or pumping attachments for added convenience.
Establish a Routine:

Incorporate pumping sessions into your daily routine at work and stick to your predetermined schedule as closely as possible. Set reminders on your phone or calendar to ensure you don't miss any pumping breaks, and communicate your schedule to your colleagues or supervisor to minimize interruptions.
Maintain Hygiene and Privacy:

Practice good hygiene by washing your hands and sterilizing your breast pump and accessories before and after each use. Use a clean surface or a pump bag to store your equipment between sessions, and avoid sharing pumping supplies with others. Maintain privacy during pumping sessions by closing the door or using a privacy screen if necessary.
Stay Flexible and Resourceful:

Be prepared to adapt your pumping schedule and location as needed based on changes in your work schedule or availability of pumping spaces. Stay flexible and resourceful in finding solutions to any challenges or obstacles you may encounter, and don't hesitate to reach out for support from your employer or colleagues.

By creating a pumping schedule and finding a private space to express milk at work, you can effectively balance your breastfeeding goals with your professional responsibilities. Remember to advocate for your needs as a breastfeeding mother and prioritize your well-being and the well-being of your baby as you navigate this important aspect of returning to work.

Maintaining Supply: Balancing Work and Breastfeeding

Balancing the demands of work with breastfeeding can present challenges, but with careful planning and dedication, it's possible to maintain a healthy milk supply while pursuing your career goals. Here are some strategies for balancing work and breastfeeding to ensure you can continue providing breast milk for your baby:

Establish a Pumping Routine:

Set a consistent pumping schedule that aligns with your work hours and your baby's feeding patterns. Aim to pump at least every 3-4 hours, or as frequently as your baby would typically nurse, to maintain your milk supply and prevent engorgement. Use a double electric breast pump for efficient and effective milk expression.
Maximize Pumping Sessions:

Make the most of your pumping sessions by ensuring you're relaxed and comfortable. Find a quiet and private space to pump, and use relaxation techniques such as deep breathing or visualization to stimulate milk flow. Massage your breasts before and during pumping to encourage milk letdown, and use breast compression to maximize milk output.
Stay Hydrated and Nourished:

Stay hydrated by drinking plenty of water throughout the day, as adequate hydration is essential for milk production. Eat a balanced diet rich in nutrient-dense foods to support your overall health and milk supply. Include foods known to promote lactation, such as oats, fenugreek, and leafy greens, in your diet.

Take Breaks to Breastfeed:

If possible, arrange your work schedule to allow for breaks to breastfeed your baby directly. Breastfeeding your baby skin-to-skin has numerous benefits for both you and your little one, including promoting bonding and boosting milk production. Take advantage of any opportunities to nurse your baby during your workday.

Store Milk Safely:

Properly store expressed breast milk in clean, labeled containers or breast milk storage bags and refrigerate or freeze it according to recommended guidelines. Label each container with the date and time of expression to ensure freshness. Transport pumped milk home in an insulated cooler bag with ice packs to keep it cold.

Communicate with Your Employer:

Openly communicate with your employer or supervisor about your breastfeeding needs and advocate for the support you require. Request flexible break times or a designated lactation room for pumping, and provide your employer with information about the benefits of supporting breastfeeding employees.

Prioritize Self-Care:

Prioritize self-care to maintain your physical and emotional well-being while juggling work and breastfeeding. Get plenty of rest, practice stress-reduction techniques such as yoga or meditation, and seek support from your partner, family, and friends. Consider joining a breastfeeding support group or online community for encouragement and advice.
Stay Flexible and Patient:

Be prepared to adjust your pumping schedule and routine as needed based on changes in your work schedule or other commitments. Stay flexible and patient with yourself as you navigate the challenges of balancing work and breastfeeding, and remember that it's okay to ask for help when you need it. By implementing these strategies and prioritizing your breastfeeding goals, you can successfully balance work and breastfeeding while maintaining a healthy milk supply for your baby. Remember that every breastfeeding journey is unique, so trust your instincts and do what works best for you and your family.

Breastfeeding is a natural and beautiful act that provides essential nourishment and comfort to your baby. However, breastfeeding in public settings can sometimes feel intimidating or uncomfortable due to societal norms or lack of support. In this chapter, we'll explore the importance of breastfeeding in public, as well as practical tips and strategies for nursing confidently wherever you are.

Normalizing Breastfeeding:

Breastfeeding is a fundamental aspect of motherhood and should be celebrated and supported in all settings. By breastfeeding in public, you help to normalize this natural behavior and empower other mothers to do the same.
Know Your Rights:

Familiarize yourself with the laws and regulations regarding breastfeeding in public in your country or region. Many places have laws that protect a mother's right to breastfeed in any location where she and her baby are authorized to be, regardless of whether it's a public or private space.
Choose Comfortable Clothing:

Wear clothing that allows for discreet and easy breastfeeding in public. Choose tops with buttons, zippers, or stretchy necklines that can be easily pulled down or lifted up for nursing. Consider investing in nursing tops or dresses with built-in nursing access for added convenience.
Practice Discreet Nursing Positions:

Experiment with different nursing positions to find ones that are comfortable and allow for discreet breastfeeding in public. Positions like the cradle hold, cross-cradle hold, or side-lying position can offer privacy while still providing optimal latch and milk flow.

Use Nursing Covers or Scarves:

If you prefer additional privacy while breastfeeding in public, consider using a nursing cover or scarf to cover yourself and your baby discreetly. Nursing covers come in a variety of styles and designs, ranging from lightweight muslin wraps to structured nursing ponchos.

Find Supportive Environments:

Seek out breastfeeding-friendly environments where you feel comfortable nursing in public. Look for cafes, restaurants, or other establishments with designated nursing areas or family-friendly facilities. Join local breastfeeding support groups or meetups to connect with other breastfeeding mothers and share experiences.

Educate and Advocate:

Educate others about the importance of breastfeeding and advocate for breastfeeding-friendly policies and practices in your community. Engage in conversations with friends, family members, and community leaders to raise awareness and promote acceptance of breastfeeding in public.

Stay Confident and Assertive:

Remember that breastfeeding is a natural and protected right, and you have every right to nurse your baby wherever you are. Trust your instincts as a mother and breastfeed with confidence, knowing that you're providing the best possible nutrition and care for your baby.

By embracing breastfeeding in public and advocating for acceptance and support, you contribute to creating a more breastfeeding-friendly culture where mothers feel empowered to nurse their babies confidently and comfortably, no matter where they are. Trust in your ability to nourish and nurture your baby, and don't let societal norms or judgments discourage you from breastfeeding in public.

Building Confidence: Overcoming the Fear of Public Breastfeeding

Breastfeeding is a beautiful and natural act that provides numerous benefits for both mother and baby. However, many breastfeeding mothers may feel apprehensive or self-conscious about nursing in public settings due to fear of judgment or discomfort. In this section, we'll explore strategies for building confidence and overcoming the fear of public breastfeeding:

Educate Yourself:

Arm yourself with knowledge about the benefits of breastfeeding and the laws protecting your right to breastfeed in public. Understanding the importance of breastfeeding and knowing your legal rights can help boost your confidence and reassure you that you're doing what's best for your baby.
Practice at Home:

Start by practicing breastfeeding in front of a mirror or with a supportive friend or family member at home. Familiarize yourself with different nursing positions and techniques so you feel more confident and comfortable when breastfeeding in public.
Start Small:

Begin by breastfeeding in public settings that feel safe and familiar, such as a friend's home or a breastfeeding support group meeting. Gradually increase your comfort level by nursing in different environments, starting with shorter outings and gradually extending the duration as you gain confidence.

Dress for Success:

Wear clothing that allows for discreet breastfeeding in public, such as tops with easy access for nursing or nursing-friendly dresses. Dressing in layers or wearing a nursing tank top under your clothes can provide additional coverage and help you feel more comfortable nursing in public.

Use Props or Accessories:

Utilize nursing covers, scarves, or baby wraps to provide privacy while breastfeeding in public. These accessories can help you feel more at ease and shield both you and your baby from prying eyes, allowing you to breastfeed with confidence wherever you are.

Focus on Your Baby:

Remember that breastfeeding is a natural and essential aspect of caring for your baby's needs. Focus on the bond you share with your little one and the joy of nourishing them with your breast milk, rather than worrying about what others may think.

Surround Yourself with Support:

Seek out supportive communities of breastfeeding mothers who can offer encouragement, advice, and solidarity. Joining a breastfeeding support group or connecting with other breastfeeding moms online can provide a valuable source of support and validation as you navigate your breastfeeding journey.

Challenge Negative Thoughts:

Challenge negative thoughts or beliefs you may have about breastfeeding in public, such as concerns about being judged or feeling embarrassed. Remind yourself that breastfeeding is a natural and normal behavior, and that you have every right to nurse your baby wherever you are.
Practice Self-Compassion:

Be kind and compassionate with yourself as you work to overcome the fear of public breastfeeding. Acknowledge any feelings of anxiety or discomfort you may experience, and give yourself permission to take things at your own pace. Celebrate each breastfeeding milestone and recognize the strength and resilience it takes to breastfeed in public.
By implementing these strategies and gradually exposing yourself to breastfeeding in public settings, you can build confidence and overcome any fears or anxieties you may have about nursing outside the home. Remember that you are not alone, and there is a supportive community of breastfeeding mothers who understand and appreciate the importance of breastfeeding in public. Trust in your abilities as a mother and embrace the beauty of breastfeeding wherever your journey takes you.

Legal Rights: Understanding Your Rights as a Breastfeeding Mother

As a breastfeeding mother, it's essential to be aware of your legal rights to breastfeed in public and in the workplace. Understanding these rights empowers you to confidently nurse your baby wherever you are without fear of discrimination or interference. Here's what you need to know about your legal rights as a breastfeeding mother:

Right to Breastfeed in Public:

In many countries and regions around the world, laws exist to protect a mother's right to breastfeed in public spaces. These laws typically stipulate that a mother can breastfeed her baby anywhere she is authorized to be, whether that's in a park, a restaurant, or a public transportation vehicle. Familiarize yourself with the specific laws and regulations in your area to ensure you understand your rights.
Anti-Discrimination Laws:

Breastfeeding discrimination is prohibited in many jurisdictions, meaning that you cannot be asked to leave a public place or denied service because you are breastfeeding. If you experience discrimination or harassment while breastfeeding in public, know that you have legal recourse to address the situation. Document the incident, if possible, and consider filing a complaint with the relevant authorities or seeking legal advice.
Workplace Protections:

In the workplace, many countries have laws that protect a mother's right to breastfeed or express breast milk while at work. These laws may include provisions for providing reasonable break time and a private, non-bathroom space for breastfeeding or pumping. Employers are generally required to accommodate breastfeeding employees and cannot discriminate against them based on their breastfeeding status.

Know Your Rights:

Educate yourself about the specific laws and regulations pertaining to breastfeeding in your country or region. Familiarize yourself with your rights as a breastfeeding mother, including any protections afforded to you in public spaces, the workplace, and other settings. Knowing your rights empowers you to advocate for yourself and confidently assert your breastfeeding rights when necessary.
Seek Support if Needed:

If you encounter any challenges or face discrimination while breastfeeding in public or in the workplace, don't hesitate to seek support from advocacy organizations, legal experts, or breastfeeding support groups. These resources can provide guidance, information, and assistance in navigating any legal issues or disputes related to breastfeeding rights.
Raise Awareness:

Help raise awareness about breastfeeding rights and advocate for positive change in your community. Share information about breastfeeding laws and rights with friends, family members, policymakers, and the general public to promote acceptance and support for breastfeeding mothers everywhere.
By understanding your legal rights as a breastfeeding mother and advocating for their protection and enforcement, you can breastfeed your baby confidently and without fear of discrimination. Remember that breastfeeding is a natural and normal behavior, and you have the right to nurse your baby wherever you are, whether at home, in public, or in the workplace.

Practical Tips: How to Nurse Discreetly in Public

Breastfeeding is a natural and beautiful act, and nursing your baby in public can be a comfortable and empowering experience with the right strategies. Here are some practical tips for nursing discreetly in public:

Choose Your Clothing Wisely:

Wear clothing that allows for easy and discreet breastfeeding. Opt for tops with buttons, zippers, or stretchy necklines that can be easily maneuvered for nursing. Dark-colored or patterned tops can also help camouflage any leaks or spills.
Use Nursing Bras and Tops:

Invest in nursing bras and tops designed specifically for breastfeeding mothers. These garments feature discreet openings or flaps that allow for easy access to the breast while providing coverage and support.
Practice at Home:

Practice breastfeeding in front of a mirror or with a supportive friend or family member at home to become more comfortable with nursing in public. Experiment with different nursing positions and techniques to find what works best for you and your baby.
Master Discreet Nursing Positions:

Learn breastfeeding positions that offer maximum coverage and privacy, such as the cradle hold, cross-cradle hold, or side-lying position. Position a nursing pillow or blanket strategically to shield both you and your baby from view while nursing.
Use Nursing Covers or Scarves:

Consider using a nursing cover, scarf, or baby wrap to provide additional privacy while breastfeeding in public. These accessories can help you feel more at ease and shield both you and your baby from prying eyes, allowing you to nurse discreetly wherever you are.

Find a Quiet Spot:

Look for quiet and comfortable places to breastfeed in public, such as a nursing room, a quiet corner of a cafe, or a designated breastfeeding area. Avoid high-traffic areas or places with distractions that may make nursing more challenging.

Practice Latch-On and Positioning:

Master the art of latching your baby onto the breast quickly and efficiently to minimize exposure. Use your clothing or a nursing cover to cover any exposed skin while your baby latches on, then adjust your clothing as needed for comfort.

Be Confident and Assertive:

Breastfeed with confidence and assert your right to nurse your baby wherever you are. Remember that breastfeeding is a natural and normal behavior, and you have the right to feed your baby in public spaces without fear of judgment or interference.

Stay Calm and Relaxed:

Keep yourself and your baby calm and relaxed while breastfeeding in public. Take deep breaths, focus on the bond you share with your baby, and try to tune out any external distractions or concerns.

By implementing these practical tips and techniques, you can nurse your baby discreetly and confidently in public, allowing you to enjoy the many benefits of breastfeeding while on the go. Trust in your abilities as a mother, and remember that breastfeeding is a beautiful and natural part of motherhood that should be celebrated and supported wherever you are
Chapter 9: Weaning Your Baby

Weaning marks the gradual transition from breastfeeding to other forms of nutrition as your baby grows and develops. While it can be an emotional and challenging journey for both you and your little one, weaning also represents an important milestone in your breastfeeding journey. In this chapter, we'll explore the process of weaning, including when and how to start, different weaning methods, and tips for a smooth transition for both you and your baby.

Understanding Weaning:

Weaning is the process of gradually reducing your baby's dependence on breast milk and introducing other sources of nutrition. It can occur naturally as your baby begins to show interest in solid foods and becomes less reliant on breastfeeding for sustenance.
Knowing When to Start:

The decision to start weaning is a personal one and can vary depending on your baby's readiness and your own preferences. Some babies may show signs of readiness for weaning around six months of age when they start showing interest in solid foods, while others may breastfeed for longer.
Gradual Transition:

Weaning is best approached gradually to minimize discomfort for both you and your baby. Begin by replacing one breastfeeding session at a time with a bottle, cup, or solid food meal, and gradually decrease the number of breastfeeding sessions over time.
Choosing the Right Method:

There are several different approaches to weaning, including baby-led weaning, mother-led weaning, and combination weaning. Choose a method that aligns with your baby's needs, preferences, and developmental stage, as well as your own comfort level and goals.
Introducing Solids:

As you begin the weaning process, introduce your baby to a variety of nutritious solid foods to complement breast milk or formula. Start with small amounts of soft, easy-to-digest foods such as pureed fruits, vegetables, and cereals, and gradually increase the texture and variety of foods as your baby becomes more comfortable with eating.
Maintaining Bonding and Comfort:

While weaning marks the end of your breastfeeding journey, it's important to find other ways to bond and comfort your baby during this transition. Offer plenty of cuddles, skin-to-skin contact, and affectionate moments to reassure your baby and strengthen your connection.
Addressing Emotional Aspects:

Weaning can be an emotional experience for both you and your baby, so be prepared for feelings of sadness, nostalgia, or guilt as you transition away from breastfeeding. Allow yourself to grieve the end of this chapter while also celebrating the milestones and achievements along the way.
Seeking Support:

Surround yourself with supportive friends, family members, and healthcare professionals who can offer guidance, encouragement, and reassurance during the weaning process. Joining a breastfeeding support group or online community can also provide valuable advice and solidarity as you navigate this journey.

By approaching weaning with patience, sensitivity, and support, you can help ensure a smooth and positive transition for both you and your baby. Remember that every breastfeeding journey is unique, and there is no one-size-fits-all approach to weaning. Trust your instincts as a parent, and prioritize your baby's well-being and comfort as you navigate this important milestone together.

Signs of Readiness: Knowing When Your Baby is Ready to Wean

Recognizing the signs that your baby is ready to begin the weaning process is an essential step in ensuring a smooth transition for both you and your little one. While the timing of weaning can vary from one baby to another, there are several common signs that may indicate your baby is ready to start the weaning journey. Here are some signs to look out for:

Interest in Solid Foods:

One of the most obvious signs that your baby is ready to start weaning is their interest in solid foods. If your baby shows curiosity about what you're eating, reaches for food, or seems eager to taste new flavors, they may be ready to begin exploring solid foods alongside breastfeeding.

Ability to Sit Up and Hold Head Steady:

As your baby develops the physical skills needed for eating solid foods, such as sitting up unassisted and holding their head steady, they may be ready to start weaning. These developmental milestones indicate that your baby has the strength and coordination to handle different textures and tastes.

Loss of Tongue Thrust Reflex:

The tongue thrust reflex is a natural reflex that babies have to push objects out of their mouths with their tongues. As this reflex diminishes, usually around six months of age, babies become better able to manage solid foods and may be ready to start weaning.

Increased Hunger and Appetite:

If your baby seems to be nursing more frequently or for shorter periods of time, it may be a sign that they are experiencing increased hunger and appetite, which could indicate readiness for solid foods. Look for cues such as rooting, smacking lips, or putting objects in their mouth, which may signal hunger.

Improved Hand-Eye Coordination:

As your baby's hand-eye coordination improves, they may become more adept at grasping objects and bringing them to their mouths. This increased coordination can make it easier for your baby to self-feed and explore different foods during the weaning process.

Decreased Interest in Breastfeeding:

While some babies continue to breastfeed enthusiastically throughout the weaning process, others may gradually lose interest in breastfeeding as they become more interested in solid foods. If your baby seems less eager to nurse or shows signs of distraction during breastfeeding sessions, it may be a sign that they are ready to start weaning.

Sleeping Through the Night:

Some babies may begin sleeping through the night or having longer stretches of sleep as they consume more calories from solid foods during the day. If your baby starts showing signs of improved sleep patterns, it may indicate that they are ready to reduce nighttime feedings and begin weaning.

Follows Your Lead:

Babies are highly attuned to their parents' behaviors and cues, so if you're modeling eating behaviors and offering solid foods during family meals, your baby may show interest in joining in. Pay attention to your baby's reactions and responses to your actions to gauge their readiness for weaning.

By observing your baby's behavior and responses, you can better understand their readiness for weaning and tailor the process to meet their needs and developmental stage. Remember that weaning is a gradual process, and it's important to be patient, responsive, and supportive as you navigate this important milestone together.

Gradual Weaning: Techniques for a Smooth Transition

Gradual weaning is a gentle and nurturing approach to transitioning your baby from breastfeeding to other forms of nutrition. By gradually reducing breastfeeding sessions and introducing alternative sources of nourishment, you can help your baby adjust to the changes while minimizing discomfort and emotional distress. Here are some techniques for achieving a smooth and gradual weaning process:

Slowly Reduce Breastfeeding Sessions:

Start by gradually reducing the number of breastfeeding sessions per day, beginning with the least preferred or least essential feeds. For example, if your baby typically nurses six times a day, consider dropping one feeding session every few days or each week until you reach your desired weaning schedule.

Replace Breastfeeds with Alternative Feedings:

As you reduce breastfeeding sessions, offer alternative forms of nourishment such as formula, expressed breast milk, or solid foods to replace the omitted feeds. Introduce these alternatives gradually and gently, allowing your baby time to adjust to the new tastes and textures.
Use Distraction Techniques:

Engage your baby in other activities or distractions during times when they would typically breastfeed to help shift their focus away from nursing. Offer toys, books, or interactive play to keep your baby occupied and satisfied without relying on breastfeeding for comfort or nourishment.
Offer Comfort and Affection:

As you reduce breastfeeding sessions, be sure to offer plenty of comfort, cuddles, and affection to reassure your baby and strengthen your bond. Spend quality time snuggling, singing, and playing together to provide emotional support during the weaning process.
Encourage Self-Feeding:

Introduce finger foods and self-feeding opportunities to encourage your baby to explore and enjoy independent eating. Offer a variety of nutritious foods in bite-sized pieces that your baby can easily grasp and bring to their mouth, allowing them to take an active role in their feeding experience.

Create New Routines and Rituals:

Establish new routines and rituals around mealtimes to help
your baby adjust to the changes in their feeding schedule.
Offer meals and snacks at consistent times throughout the
day, and create a calm and relaxed environment for eating to
promote positive associations with food.
Be Patient and Flexible:

Remember that weaning is a gradual process that unfolds at
your baby's pace, so be patient and flexible as you navigate
the journey together. Allow your baby time to adjust to the
changes, and be responsive to their cues and needs
throughout the weaning process.
Seek Support and Guidance:

If you encounter challenges or concerns during the weaning
process, don't hesitate to seek support and guidance from
healthcare professionals, lactation consultants, or
breastfeeding support groups. They can offer valuable advice,
encouragement, and reassurance to help you navigate the
transition with confidence and ease.
By implementing these techniques for gradual weaning, you
can help ensure a smooth and positive transition for both you
and your baby as you navigate this important milestone
together. Remember to trust your instincts as a parent, and
prioritize your baby's well-being and comfort throughout the
weaning process.

Emotional Aspects: Coping with the End of Breastfeeding

The end of breastfeeding can evoke a range of emotions for both mother and baby, marking the conclusion of a significant chapter in your breastfeeding journey. While weaning is a natural and necessary transition, it's normal to experience a mix of emotions, including sadness, nostalgia, relief, and even guilt. Here are some strategies for coping with the emotional aspects of weaning:

Acknowledge Your Feelings:

Allow yourself to acknowledge and express your feelings about the end of breastfeeding without judgment. Recognize that it's okay to feel sad or nostalgic about the transition, even if you're also feeling relieved or ready to move on.
Give Yourself Time to Grieve:

It's natural to grieve the end of breastfeeding, especially if it's been an important and rewarding experience for you. Give yourself permission to mourn the loss of this special bond and acknowledge the significance of the journey you've shared with your baby.
Celebrate Milestones and Achievements:

Take time to celebrate the milestones and achievements you've reached during your breastfeeding journey, whether it's nursing for a certain length of time, overcoming challenges, or nurturing a strong bond with your baby. Reflect on the positive memories and experiences you've shared together.

Focus on the Benefits of Weaning:

While it's normal to mourn the end of breastfeeding, try to focus on the positive aspects of weaning and the new opportunities it brings for both you and your baby. Remind yourself of the freedom and flexibility that comes with weaning, as well as the exciting developmental milestones ahead.

Stay Connected with Your Baby:

Find other ways to nurture and bond with your baby beyond breastfeeding. Spend quality time cuddling, playing, and engaging in activities together to maintain and strengthen your connection. Remember that breastfeeding is just one of many ways to nurture your baby's emotional and physical well-being.

Seek Support and Understanding:

Reach out to friends, family members, or other mothers who have experienced weaning for support and understanding during this emotional time. Sharing your feelings with others who can empathize with your experience can provide comfort and validation.

Practice Self-Care:

Take care of yourself emotionally and physically during the weaning process by prioritizing self-care activities that nourish your mind, body, and spirit. Engage in activities that bring you joy and relaxation, such as exercise, hobbies, or spending time in nature.

Trust Your Instincts:

Trust your instincts as a mother and prioritize what feels right for you and your baby as you navigate the emotional aspects of weaning. Listen to your inner voice and follow your intuition as you make decisions about the weaning process. Remember that every breastfeeding journey is unique, and there is no one-size-fits-all approach to coping with the end of breastfeeding. Be gentle with yourself and give yourself the time and space you need to process your feelings and embrace this new chapter in your relationship with your baby.

Breastfeeding is a deeply personal and individual experience, and there are certain special circumstances that may arise during the breastfeeding journey that require unique considerations and approaches. In this chapter, we'll explore some of these special circumstances and provide guidance and support for navigating them with confidence and compassion.

Multiples or Preterm Babies:

Parents of multiples or preterm babies may face unique challenges when it comes to breastfeeding, such as coordinating feeding schedules, establishing milk supply, and ensuring each baby receives adequate nourishment. We'll discuss strategies for breastfeeding multiples or preterm infants, including tandem feeding, paced feeding, and seeking support from lactation consultants or support groups. Breastfeeding after Breast Surgery:

Women who have undergone breast surgery, such as breast reduction or augmentation, may encounter challenges with breastfeeding due to changes in breast tissue and milk ducts. We'll explore techniques for maximizing milk production, working with a lactation consultant to address breastfeeding difficulties, and supplementing breastfeeding with alternative feeding methods if necessary.
Medical Conditions and Medications:

Certain medical conditions or medications may impact breastfeeding, either by affecting milk production or posing potential risks to the baby. We'll provide information on navigating breastfeeding with common medical conditions such as diabetes, thyroid disorders, or PCOS, as well as guidelines for safely breastfeeding while taking medications.
Relactation and Induced Lactation:

Some mothers may wish to relactate or induce lactation after a period of weaning or if they did not breastfeed initially. We'll discuss strategies for relactation, including frequent breastfeeding

or pumping, skin-to-skin contact, and herbal supplements, as well as techniques for inducing lactation in adoptive or surrogate mothers.
Breastfeeding Challenges and Complications:

Breastfeeding may not always go as smoothly as expected, and parents may encounter challenges such as engorgement, mastitis, nipple pain, or low milk supply. We'll offer practical tips and advice for managing common breastfeeding complications, including seeking professional support from lactation consultants or healthcare providers.
Weaning and Transitioning to Solids:

Transitioning from breastfeeding to solid foods is a significant milestone for both mother and baby. We'll explore strategies for gentle weaning, introducing solids, and ensuring adequate nutrition during the transition period, as well as tips for managing emotions and navigating changes in the breastfeeding relationship.

By addressing these special circumstances with empathy, understanding, and practical guidance, we can empower parents to overcome challenges and continue their breastfeeding journey with confidence and resilience. Remember that every breastfeeding experience is unique, and there is no one-size-fits-all solution. Trust your instincts as a parent, seek support when needed, and prioritize the well-being of both you and your baby as you navigate these special circumstances together.

Tandem Nursing: Breastfeeding Multiples or Siblings

Tandem nursing, the practice of breastfeeding two or more children of different ages simultaneously, can be a rewarding and fulfilling experience for both mother and children. Whether you're nursing twins, siblings close in age, or a combination of both, tandem nursing presents unique challenges and benefits. Here's a guide to navigating tandem nursing with confidence and ease:

Establishing a Routine:

Establishing a routine that works for both you and your children is essential for successful tandem nursing. Consider factors such as each child's feeding schedule, preferences, and individual needs when planning your nursing sessions.

Positioning and Latching:

Experiment with different nursing positions to find what works best for tandem nursing. Positions such as the football hold, cradle hold, or side-lying position may be particularly helpful for nursing two children at once. Ensure each child has a good latch and is comfortable during feedings.

Managing Milk Supply:

Tandem nursing can place additional demands on your milk supply, especially when breastfeeding multiple children. To maintain an adequate milk supply, ensure you're staying well-hydrated, eating a nutritious diet, and nursing frequently. Utilize breast compression techniques and switch sides regularly to encourage milk flow.
Balancing Attention and Bonding:

One of the benefits of tandem nursing is the opportunity to bond with each of your children individually while still meeting their breastfeeding needs. Take advantage of nursing sessions to connect with each child, offer cuddles, and enjoy quiet moments together.
Addressing Sibling Rivalry:

Sibling rivalry and jealousy may arise when tandem nursing, especially if one child is older than the other. Be mindful of each child's emotional needs and offer reassurance, attention, and affection to help foster a positive sibling relationship.
Seeking Support:

Tandem nursing can be physically and emotionally demanding, so don't hesitate to seek support from your partner, family members, or breastfeeding support groups. Connecting with other mothers who have experience with tandem nursing can provide valuable advice, encouragement, and camaraderie.
Self-Care and Boundaries:

Prioritize self-care and set boundaries to ensure you're taking care of your own physical and emotional well-being. Practice self-care activities such as rest, relaxation, and engaging in hobbies or activities that bring you joy and fulfillment.
Flexibility and Patience:

Remember that tandem nursing is a journey, and it's okay to adapt and adjust your approach as needed. Be patient with yourself and your children as you navigate the challenges and joys of breastfeeding multiples or siblings.

Tandem nursing is a beautiful expression of maternal love and nurturing that can strengthen the bond between you and your children. By embracing the unique joys and challenges of tandem nursing, you can create a nurturing and supportive breastfeeding relationship that benefits both you and your little one

Nursing Through Pregnancy: What to Expect

Nursing through pregnancy, also known as tandem nursing during pregnancy, is the practice of breastfeeding a child while pregnant with another. This journey can be both rewarding and challenging, with unique considerations for both the breastfeeding child and the expectant mother. Here's what to expect when nursing through pregnancy:

Changes in Milk Supply and Sensitivity:

During pregnancy, hormonal changes can affect milk production and composition, leading to fluctuations in milk supply and changes in the taste and composition of breast milk. Some nursing mothers may experience a decrease in milk supply or nipple sensitivity, while others may continue to produce milk normally.

Nursing Aversion and Discomfort:

Some breastfeeding mothers may experience nursing aversion or discomfort during pregnancy, characterized by feelings of irritation, agitation, or aversion while breastfeeding. This can be attributed to hormonal changes, increased sensitivity, or changes in the breastfeeding child's nursing behavior.

Child's Response to Pregnancy:

Nursing through pregnancy can evoke various responses from the breastfeeding child, ranging from continued nursing as usual to decreased interest in breastfeeding or self-weaning. Children may pick up on changes in milk supply or sensitivity and adjust their nursing frequency or behavior accordingly.
Nutritional Considerations:

Breastfeeding during pregnancy requires careful attention to maternal and child nutrition to ensure adequate nourishment for both mother and breastfeeding child. Expectant mothers should prioritize a balanced diet rich in essential nutrients, vitamins, and minerals to support both pregnancy and breastfeeding.
Physical and Emotional Well-being:

Nursing through pregnancy can be physically and emotionally demanding for the expectant mother, especially as pregnancy progresses. It's essential to prioritize self-care, rest, and relaxation to support maternal well-being and energy levels during this time.
Communication with Healthcare Providers:

Expectant mothers who choose to nurse through pregnancy should communicate openly with their healthcare providers about their breastfeeding plans and any concerns or challenges they may encounter. Healthcare providers can offer guidance, support, and resources to help navigate the unique considerations of nursing during pregnancy.
Preparing for Tandem Nursing:

Nursing through pregnancy may lead to tandem nursing once the new baby is born. Expectant mothers should prepare for tandem nursing by educating themselves about breastfeeding techniques, positioning, and managing the needs of both children simultaneously.

Embracing the Journey:
Nursing through pregnancy is a deeply personal and
individual experience that varies from woman to woman and
child to child. Embrace the journey with patience, compassion,
and an open mind, trusting your instincts as a mother and
prioritizing the well-being of both yourself and your
breastfeeding child.
Nursing through pregnancy is a testament to the unique bond
between mother and child, offering comfort, nourishment,
and connection during a time of profound physical and
emotional changes. By understanding what to expect and
embracing the journey with an open heart, expectant mothers
can navigate the challenges and joys of nursing through
pregnancy with confidence and grace.

Breastfeeding Preemies: Special Considerations for Premature
Infants

Breastfeeding a premature infant, or preemie, presents unique
challenges and considerations. Premature babies, born before
37 weeks of gestation, often have special nutritional needs and
require additional support to thrive. Here's what you need to
know about breastfeeding a preemie:

Benefits of Breast Milk for Preemies:

Breast milk is particularly beneficial for preemies, providing
essential nutrients, antibodies, and growth factors that
support their development and immune system. It helps
protect against infections, promotes brain development, and
improves overall health outcomes.
Establishing Milk Supply:

For mothers of preemies, establishing and maintaining a milk supply is crucial. Frequent pumping, ideally every 2-3 hours, can help stimulate milk production. Using a hospital-grade breast pump and practicing skin-to-skin contact (kangaroo care) can also boost milk supply.
NICU Support:

Neonatal Intensive Care Units (NICUs) often have lactation consultants and staff who specialize in supporting breastfeeding mothers. They can provide guidance on pumping, milk storage, and transitioning to direct breastfeeding when the baby is ready.
Feeding Challenges:

Preemies may face challenges such as weak suck reflexes, fatigue, and difficulty latching. These issues often improve as the baby grows and develops. Initially, feeding may involve a combination of tube feeding, bottle feeding with expressed milk, and eventually direct breastfeeding.
Use of Breast Milk Fortifiers:

Sometimes, breast milk fortifiers are added to expressed breast milk to meet the higher nutritional needs of preemies. These fortifiers provide additional calories, protein, and nutrients essential for their growth and development.
Transitioning to Breastfeeding:

As preemies grow stronger, they can begin to transition from tube or bottle feeding to breastfeeding. This process involves patience and gradual steps, such as practicing non-nutritive sucking (letting the baby suck at the breast after pumping) and offering the breast when the baby is calm and alert.
Kangaroo Care:

Kangaroo care, or skin-to-skin contact, is highly beneficial for preemies. It helps regulate their body temperature, heart rate, and breathing, and promotes bonding. This practice also supports breastfeeding by encouraging natural breastfeeding instincts.
Patience and Persistence:

Breastfeeding a preemie requires patience, persistence, and flexibility. Celebrate small successes and understand that progress may be gradual. Every drop of breast milk you provide is valuable, whether through direct breastfeeding or pumping.
Support Systems:

Building a strong support system is essential. Engage with lactation consultants, NICU staff, and support groups for mothers of preemies. Sharing experiences and receiving encouragement can be incredibly helpful during this challenging journey.
Monitoring Growth and Development:

Regular follow-ups with healthcare providers are crucial to monitor your preemie's growth and development. They will assess weight gain, feeding progress, and overall health to ensure that your baby is thriving.
Breastfeeding a preemie is a unique journey that requires dedication, resilience, and support. While it may present challenges, the rewards of providing your preemie with breast milk are immense. By understanding the special considerations and seeking the right support, you can navigate this journey with confidence and provide your preemie with the best possible start in life.

Maintaining health and wellness is crucial for both the breastfeeding mother and her baby. This chapter provides comprehensive insights into the key aspects of health and wellness during the breastfeeding journey.

Maternal Health
1. Postpartum Recovery:
Physical Recovery: Tips for healing after childbirth, including managing pain, dealing with postpartum bleeding, and getting enough rest.
Emotional Recovery: Recognizing and managing postpartum depression and anxiety. Importance of seeking support and professional help when needed.
2. Nutritional Needs:
Balanced Diet: Importance of a well-rounded diet rich in fruits, vegetables, whole grains, and lean proteins to support milk production and overall health.
Supplements: Discussing the need for continued prenatal vitamins, especially those containing iron, calcium, and DHA.
Hydration: Ensuring adequate fluid intake to maintain milk supply and overall health.
3. Physical Activity:
Exercise Guidelines: Safe ways to incorporate physical activity postpartum, including gentle exercises like walking, yoga, and pelvic floor exercises.
Benefits of Exercise: How regular physical activity can boost energy levels, improve mood, and aid in postpartum recovery.
Infant Health
1. Monitoring Growth and Development:
Growth Charts: Understanding percentiles and growth curves used by pediatricians to track your baby's growth.

Developmental Milestones: Key milestones to expect in the first year, from motor skills to cognitive and social development.

2. Immunizations and Check-Ups:

Vaccination Schedule: Overview of recommended vaccines and the importance of adhering to the vaccination schedule.

Regular Check-Ups: Importance of routine pediatric visits to monitor growth, development, and address any concerns.

3. Common Infant Ailments:

Colic: Understanding and managing colic, including soothing techniques and dietary adjustments.

Reflux: Identifying and managing reflux symptoms, and when to seek medical advice.

Fevers and Infections: Recognizing signs of illness and understanding when to seek medical care.

Mental Wellness

1. Managing Stress:

Stress Reduction Techniques: Mindfulness, meditation, and relaxation exercises that can help manage stress and promote emotional well-being.

Self-Care: Importance of taking time for self-care activities, such as hobbies, socializing, and relaxation.

2. Building a Support Network:

Family and Friends: Leveraging support from family and friends for practical help and emotional support.

Support Groups: Joining breastfeeding or new parent support groups for shared experiences and advice.

3. Professional Help:

Lactation Consultants: When and how to seek help from lactation consultants for breastfeeding issues.

Mental Health Professionals: Recognizing when to seek professional help for mental health concerns, such as postpartum depression or anxiety.

Sleep and Rest

1. Importance of Sleep:

For Mothers: Strategies for maximizing sleep and rest, including napping when the baby sleeps and sharing nighttime duties.

For Babies: Creating a safe sleep environment and establishing healthy sleep habits for your baby.

2. Sleep Challenges:

Newborn Sleep Patterns: Understanding normal newborn sleep patterns and how to cope with frequent night wakings.

Safe Sleep Practices: Guidelines for reducing the risk of SIDS (sudden infant death syndrome), including back sleeping and a safe crib environment.

Conclusion

Maintaining health and wellness is a dynamic and ongoing process that encompasses physical, emotional, and mental well-being for both mother and baby. By prioritizing these aspects and seeking support when needed, you can navigate the breastfeeding journey with greater ease and confidence. Remember, taking care of yourself is just as important as caring for your baby, and a healthy, happy mother is the foundation for a thriving baby.

Recognizing Illness: When You or Your Baby is Sick

For the mother

**1. Common Postpartum Illnesses:

Mastitis: Symptoms include breast pain, redness, and fever. Prompt treatment is crucial to prevent complications.

Postpartum Infections: Look for signs such as fever, chills, and unusual discharge, and seek medical advice if these occur.

Thyroid Issues: Postpartum thyroiditis can cause fatigue, weight changes, and mood swings. Monitoring thyroid levels is important if symptoms arise.

**2. Symptoms to Watch For:

Fever: A fever above 100.4°F (38°C) warrants medical attention.

Severe Pain: Unusual or severe pain in the abdomen, breasts, or pelvic area should be evaluated.
Mental Health Concerns: Symptoms of postpartum depression or anxiety, such as persistent sadness, loss of interest in activities, or extreme worry, should be addressed with a healthcare provider.
**3. When to Seek Help:

Emergency Situations: Seek immediate medical attention for symptoms such as heavy bleeding, severe abdominal pain, or high fever.
Persistent Symptoms: If symptoms like fatigue, pain, or mood changes persist, consult your healthcare provider for further evaluation and support.
For the Baby
**1. Recognizing Common Infant Illnesses:

Fevers: A fever in an infant under three months old is a medical emergency. For older infants, monitor for additional symptoms and seek advice if the fever persists.
Colds and Respiratory Infections: Symptoms include congestion, coughing, and difficulty feeding. Seek medical advice if your baby has trouble breathing, is very irritable, or has a high fever.
Ear Infections: Look for signs such as ear pulling, fussiness, and fever. Ear infections are common and often require medical treatment.
**2. Signs of Serious Illness:

Lethargy: A baby who is unusually sleepy or difficult to wake should be seen by a doctor.
Dehydration: Symptoms include fewer wet diapers, a dry mouth, and sunken eyes. Ensure your baby is getting enough fluids and seek medical help if dehydration is suspected.
Rashes: While many rashes are harmless, seek medical advice if a rash is accompanied by fever or if it spreads rapidly.

3. When to Call the Doctor:

Feeding Issues: Difficulty feeding, persistent vomiting, or poor weight gain are reasons to contact your healthcare provider.
Breathing Problems: Rapid breathing, wheezing, or blue-tinged skin are signs of respiratory distress and require immediate attention.
Behavioral Changes: Unusual irritability, excessive crying, or lack of responsiveness should be evaluated promptly.
4. Preparing for Doctor Visits:

Keep a Symptom Diary: Document symptoms, including their onset, frequency, and severity. This information can help your healthcare provider make an accurate diagnosis.
Know Your Baby's Medical History: Be prepared to discuss your baby's feeding patterns, sleep habits, and any previous illnesses or medical conditions.
Stay Calm: Approach doctor visits with a calm demeanor to help keep your baby relaxed. Remember that seeking help is a crucial part of ensuring your baby's health and well-being.
Conclusion
Recognizing the signs of illness in both yourself and your baby is crucial for timely intervention and treatment. By understanding common symptoms and knowing when to seek medical help, you can protect your health and that of your baby. Remember, it's always better to consult with a healthcare provider if you have any concerns about your or your baby's health. Your vigilance and proactive care are key components of a healthy breastfeeding journey.

Medications and Breastfeeding: What's Safe and What to Avoid
Understanding Medication Safety

**1. Consulting Healthcare Providers:

Before Taking Any Medication: Always consult your healthcare provider or a lactation consultant before taking any medication, including over-the-counter drugs, supplements, and herbal remedies.
Discuss Your Breastfeeding Status: Make sure your healthcare provider knows you are breastfeeding so they can prescribe the safest options.
**2. Categories of Medication Safety:

Safe: Medications that are considered safe for breastfeeding mothers and their babies.
Use with Caution: Medications that require careful monitoring or may be safe under certain conditions.
Avoid: Medications that are known to be harmful to breastfeeding infants.
Safe Medications
**1. Pain Relievers:

Acetaminophen (Tylenol): Generally considered safe for breastfeeding mothers.
Ibuprofen (Advil, Motrin): Also deemed safe and effective for pain relief.
**2. Antibiotics:

Penicillin's and Cephalosporins: These classes of antibiotics are usually safe for breastfeeding mothers.
Erythromycin: Often considered a safe alternative if penicillin's are not suitable.
**3. Allergy Medications:

Antihistamines (Loratadine, Cetirizine): Non-drowsy antihistamines are typically safe.
**4. Vaccinations:

Most Vaccines: Including the flu shot and Tdap, are safe and recommended for breastfeeding mothers.

Medications to Use with Caution

**1. Antidepressants:

Selective Serotonin Reuptake Inhibitors (SSRIs): Some, like sertraline (Zoloft), are considered safer options.

Consultation Required: Always discuss with your healthcare provider to determine the best option and monitor your baby for any adverse effects.

**2. Cold and Cough Remedies:

Decongestants (Pseudoephedrine): Can reduce milk supply; use only if necessary and under medical guidance.

Cough Suppressants (Dextromethorphan): Generally safe but should be used minimally.

**3. Herbal Supplements:

Limited Research: Many herbal supplements lack sufficient research on their safety for breastfeeding mothers. Always consult with your healthcare provider before use.

Medications to Avoid

**1. Certain Pain Medications:

Aspirin: Can cause Reye's syndrome in infants and should be avoided.

Codeine and Tramadol: Risk of serious side effects in infants, including difficulty breathing.

**2. Chemotherapy Drugs:

Contraindicated: These medications are generally not safe for breastfeeding mothers.

**3. Radioactive Iodine:

For Thyroid Conditions: Should be avoided due to the risk of transferring harmful radiation to the baby.

**4. Recreational Drugs:

Substances like Marijuana and Cocaine: Should be strictly avoided due to harmful effects on the baby.
Practical Tips for Medication Use
**1. Timing Doses:

Breastfeeding Schedule: Take medications right after breastfeeding to minimize the baby's exposure to the drug when it is at its peak concentration in your bloodstream.
**2. Monitoring Your Baby:

Watch for Side Effects: Look for signs of adverse reactions in your baby, such as unusual sleepiness, irritability, feeding difficulties, or rash.
**3. Stay Informed:

Use Reliable Resources: Refer to reputable sources like the LactMed database, which provides up-to-date information on the safety of various medications during breastfeeding.
**4. Seek Professional Guidance:

Lactation Consultants: They can offer specific advice and support for managing medications while breastfeeding.
Conclusion
Navigating medication use while breastfeeding can be challenging, but with the right information and professional guidance, you can make safe choices for both you and your baby. Always consult with your healthcare provider before starting any new medication, and stay vigilant for any changes in your baby's behavior or health. Your commitment to staying informed and cautious will help ensure a healthy breastfeeding journey.

Self-Care: Maintaining Your Own Health and Well-being

The Importance of Self-Care
**1. Why Self-Care Matters:

Physical Health: Taking care of your body ensures you have the energy and stamina needed for breastfeeding and daily activities.
Mental Health: Managing stress and emotional well-being is crucial for a positive breastfeeding experience.
Modeling Healthy Behaviors: Demonstrating self-care sets a positive example for your child and reinforces the importance of personal health.
Physical Self-Care
**1. Rest and Sleep:

Prioritize Sleep: Aim for restful sleep whenever possible, taking naps when your baby sleeps.
Create a Sleep-Conducive Environment: Ensure your bedroom is comfortable, dark, and quiet.
**2. Nutrition:
Balanced Diet: Eat a variety of foods to ensure you're getting essential nutrients.
Regular Meals: Don't skip meals; opt for nutrient-dense snacks if you're short on time.
Hydration: Drink plenty of water to stay hydrated and support milk production.
**3. Exercise:

Stay Active: Engage in moderate exercise like walking, yoga, or postpartum fitness classes.
Listen to Your Body: Adjust your activity level based on how you feel and any guidance from your healthcare provider.
Mental and Emotional Self-Care
**1. Managing Stress:

Mindfulness and Meditation: Practice mindfulness or meditation to reduce stress and increase relaxation.

Breathing Exercises: Use deep breathing techniques to calm your mind and body.
**2. Emotional Support:

Talk to Someone: Share your feelings and experiences with a partner, friend, or support group.
Professional Help: Don't hesitate to seek help from a therapist or counselor if you're feeling overwhelmed or anxious.
**3. Time for Yourself:

Personal Time: Schedule regular "me-time" for activities you enjoy, such as reading, hobbies, or taking a bath.
Boundaries: Set boundaries to ensure you have time and space for self-care without feeling guilty.
Practical Self-Care Tips
**1. Creating a Routine:

Daily Routine: Establish a routine that includes time for meals, rest, and relaxation.
Flexibility: Be adaptable and allow your routine to change as needed.
**2. Utilizing Support Systems:

Delegate Tasks: Share responsibilities with your partner or family members.
Accept Help: Be open to accepting help from friends and family, whether it's cooking meals or babysitting.
**3. Staying Connected:

Social Interaction: Maintain connections with friends and loved ones to prevent feelings of isolation.
Online Communities: Join breastfeeding and parenting groups online for support and advice.
Long-term Self-Care Strategies
**1. Ongoing Learning:

Stay Informed: Continue to educate yourself about breastfeeding and postpartum health.
Seek Resources: Use books, articles, and online courses to expand your knowledge.
**2. Regular Check-ups:

Healthcare Appointments: Keep up with regular health check-ups for both you and your baby.
Postpartum Care: Attend all postpartum visits and address any concerns with your healthcare provider.
**3. Adjusting Self-Care Practices:

Evolving Needs: Recognize that your self-care needs will change over time and adjust your practices accordingly.
Reflect and Adapt: Regularly reflect on what's working and what's not, making necessary changes to your self-care routine.
Conclusion
Maintaining your health and well-being through self-care is essential for a positive breastfeeding experience and overall postpartum recovery. By prioritizing rest, nutrition, exercise, emotional health, and support systems, you can nurture both yourself and your baby effectively. Remember, self-care is not a luxury but a necessity, and taking care of yourself will enable you to be the best parent you can be.

The Importance of a Support Network
1. Emotional Support:

Sharing Experiences: Talking to others who understand what you're going through can provide comfort and reduce feelings of isolation.
Empathy and Understanding: Friends, family, and other mothers can offer empathy and understanding during challenging times.
2. Practical Assistance:

Help with Daily Tasks: A support network can assist with household chores, meal preparation, and childcare, giving you more time to rest and recover.
Childcare Relief: Trusted friends and family can provide occasional childcare, allowing you time for self-care or to run errands.
3. Informational Support:

Advice and Tips: Experienced mothers and healthcare professionals can offer valuable advice and tips on breastfeeding and newborn care.
Resource Sharing: Your network can share resources such as books, articles, and local support groups that may be beneficial.
Types of Support Networks
1. Family and Friends:

Immediate Family: Partners, parents, siblings, and close relatives can provide direct and immediate support.
Friends: Close friends, especially those who are parents, can offer practical advice and emotional support.

2. Professional Support:

Healthcare Providers: Doctors, lactation consultants, and nurses can provide expert guidance and medical support.
Therapists and Counselors: Mental health professionals can help manage stress, anxiety, and postpartum depression.
3. Community and Online Support:

Local Support Groups: Parenting and breastfeeding support groups in your community offer a space to share experiences and receive support.
Online Communities: Social media groups, forums, and online support networks provide access to a broader community of mothers and experts.
Building Your Support Network
1. Identifying Your Needs:

Assess Your Needs: Determine what kind of support you need most, whether it's emotional, practical, or informational.
Prioritize: Focus on building a network that meets your highest priorities first.
2. Reaching Out:

Communicate: Don't hesitate to reach out to friends, family, and professionals for support. Be clear about your needs and how they can help.
Join Groups: Participate in local and online support groups to connect with other mothers and experts.
3. Creating a Plan:
Organize Your Network: Make a list of your support network, including contact information and how each person can help.
Establish Routines: Set regular check-ins with your support network, such as weekly calls with friends or monthly visits with a therapist.
Maintaining Your Support Network

1. Regular Communication:
Stay Connected: Keep in regular contact with your support network through calls, texts, and meet-ups.
Share Updates: Keep your network informed about your progress, challenges, and any changes in your needs.
2. Offering Support in Return:

Reciprocate: Support is a two-way street. Offer help to others in your network when they need it.
Express Gratitude: Show appreciation for the support you receive through thank-you note, small gestures, and verbal acknowledgment.
3. Adjusting as Needed:

Reevaluate Needs: Periodically reassess your needs and make adjustments to your support network as necessary.
Seek New Resources: Don't be afraid to seek new resources or replace support systems that are no longer effective.
Tips for Building a Strong Support Network
**1. Be Open and Honest:

Share Your Feelings: Open up about your experiences, emotions, and challenges to build deeper connections.
Ask for Help: Don't be afraid to ask for help when you need it.
**2. Utilize Technology:

Stay Connected Online: Use social media, messaging apps, and video calls to stay connected with your support network, especially if they're not nearby.
Access Resources: Take advantage of online resources, such as virtual support groups and telehealth services.

**3. Participate Actively:
Engage in Groups: Actively participate in support groups by attending meetings, contributing to discussions, and offering support to others.

Seek Professional Help: Don't hesitate to seek professional help when needed, whether it's a lactation consultant, a therapist, or a healthcare provider.

Conclusion

Building a strong support network is crucial for a successful and positive breastfeeding experience. By surrounding yourself with supportive family, friends, professionals, and community resources, you can navigate the challenges of breastfeeding and motherhood with confidence. Remember, seeking and accepting support is a sign of strength, and it will help you provide the best care for your baby while taking care of yourself.

Finding Support Groups: Connecting with Other Breastfeeding Mothers

1. Importance of Support Groups

1. Emotional Support:

Shared Experiences: Support groups offer a space to share your experiences with others who understand what you're going through.

Empathy and Understanding: Fellow mothers can provide empathy, understanding, and encouragement, making you feel less isolated.

2. Practical Advice:

Breastfeeding Tips: Learn practical tips and techniques for breastfeeding from experienced mothers.

Problem-Solving: Get help troubleshooting common breastfeeding issues such as latching problems, sore nipples, and milk supply concerns.

3. Information and Resources:

Educational Resources: Access to a wealth of information on breastfeeding, baby care, and parenting.

Expert Guidance: Many support groups have lactation consultants or healthcare professionals who can provide expert advice.
2. Types of Support Groups
1. In-Person Support Groups:

Local Community Groups: Many communities have local breastfeeding support groups that meet regularly.
Healthcare Provider Groups: Some hospitals and clinics offer breastfeeding support groups led by lactation consultants or nurses.
2. Online Support Groups:

Social media: Platforms like Facebook have numerous breastfeeding support groups where you can connect with other mothers.
Parenting Forums: Websites such as BabyCenter, La Leche League, and What to Expect have forums dedicated to breastfeeding support.
Virtual Meetings: Some support groups offer virtual meetings via Zoom or other video conferencing tools.
3. How to Find Support Groups
1. Ask Your Healthcare Provider:

Recommendations: Ask your doctor, midwife, or lactation consultant for recommendations on local breastfeeding support groups.
Hospital Resources: Inquire about support groups offered by the hospital where you gave birth.
2. Research Online:

Google Search: Perform a search for breastfeeding support groups in your area.
Support Organization Websites: Visit websites of organizations like La Leche League, which has a directory of local chapters and support groups.

3. Community Resources:
Community Centers: Check with community centers, libraries, and local health departments for information on support groups.
Parenting Classes: Attend parenting classes or prenatal classes that often provide information on local support resources.
4. Social Media and Apps:

Facebook Groups: Join Facebook groups dedicated to breastfeeding support.
Parenting Apps: Use apps like Peanut or BabyCenter that connect you with local and online breastfeeding support communities.
4. Joining and Participating in Support Groups
1. Attend Meetings:

In-Person: If possible, attend in-person meetings to build stronger connections with other mothers.
Virtual: Participate in virtual meetings if in-person attendance is not feasible.
2. Engage Actively:

Share Your Story: Share your breastfeeding journey, challenges, and successes with the group.
Ask Questions: Don't hesitate to ask for advice or help with specific breastfeeding issues.
3. Offer Support:

Encourage Others: Offer encouragement and support to other mothers in the group.
Share Tips: Share any tips or techniques that have worked for you.
4. Utilize Resources:

Educational Materials: Take advantage of any educational materials or resources provided by the group.

Expert Advice: Utilize the expertise of lactation consultants or healthcare professionals who may be part of the group.
5. Building Lasting Connections
1. Stay in Touch:

Exchange Contact Information: Exchange contact information with other mothers to stay in touch outside of group meetings.
Create Sub-Groups: Form smaller sub-groups with mothers who share similar experiences or challenges.
2. Plan Social Activities:

Playdates: Organize playdates for your babies to foster connections.
Mother's Meetups: Plan social meetups for mothers to relax and share experiences in a more casual setting.
3. Continue Participation:

Regular Attendance: Make attending support group meetings a regular part of your routine.
Long-Term Engagement: Continue engaging with the group even after you have overcome initial breastfeeding challenges to support new mothers.
Conclusion
Finding and participating in breastfeeding support groups can significantly enhance your breastfeeding experience. These groups provide a community of understanding, practical advice, and valuable resources, helping you navigate the journey of breastfeeding with confidence. By connecting with other breastfeeding mothers, you can share experiences, overcome challenges, and build lasting friendships that support both you and your baby.

Professional Help: When to Seek Advice from a Lactation Consultant
1. Understanding the Role of a Lactation Consultant
1. Expertise in Breastfeeding:

Specialized Training: Lactation consultants have specialized training in breastfeeding support and management.
Certified Professionals: Many are certified through organizations like the International Board of Lactation Consultant Examiners (IBLCE).
2. Comprehensive Support:

Personalized Assistance: They provide personalized assistance tailored to your specific needs and challenges.
Evidence-Based Guidance: They offer evidence-based guidance to ensure the best breastfeeding practices.
2. When to Seek Professional Help
1. Difficulty with Latching:

Painful Latch: If breastfeeding is consistently painful, it may indicate an issue with the latch.
Baby's Difficulty: If your baby has trouble latching onto the breast or frequently loses the latch.
2. Low Milk Supply:

Insufficient Output: If you're concerned that you're not producing enough milk to meet your baby's needs.
Feeding Frequency: If your baby is not gaining weight as expected or seems hungry after most feedings.
3. Breast Pain and Nipple Issues:

Persistent Pain: Ongoing pain during or between feedings, cracked or bleeding nipples, or other nipple trauma.
Breast Infections: Signs of mastitis or breast infections, such as redness, swelling, warmth, or flu-like symptoms.
4. Baby's Weight Gain and Feeding Issues:

Slow Weight Gain: If your baby is not gaining weight as expected or is losing weight.

Feeding Duration: If feedings are consistently very short (less than 10 minutes) or very long (more than an hour) without satisfaction.
5. Breastfeeding Multiples:

Tandem Nursing: If you are breastfeeding twins, triplets, or more, and need strategies for managing feedings.
Feeding Schedules: Help with creating and managing feeding schedules for multiple babies.
6. Premature or Special Needs Babies:

Preterm Babies: If your baby was born prematurely and you need specialized techniques for feeding.
Special Conditions: If your baby has medical conditions that affect breastfeeding, such as a cleft palate or tongue-tie.
7. Returning to Work:

Pumping Strategies: If you need help establishing a pumping routine to maintain milk supply.
Milk Storage: Advice on storing and transporting breast milk.
8. Emotional and Psychological Support:

Stress and Anxiety: If breastfeeding challenges are causing significant stress or anxiety.
Postpartum Depression: If you are experiencing symptoms of postpartum depression or anxiety.
3. How to Find a Lactation Consultant
1. Healthcare Provider Referral:

Ask Your Doctor: Ask your obstetrician, pediatrician, or family doctor for recommendations.
Hospital Services: Many hospitals have lactation consultants on staff who can assist you.
2. Professional Organizations:

IBLCE Directory: Use the International Board of Lactation
Consultant Examiners (IBLCE) directory to find certified
consultants.
La Leche League: Contact La Leche League for referrals to
local lactation consultants.
3. Community Resources:

Breastfeeding Support Groups: Local support groups often
have information on reputable lactation consultants.
Parenting Classes: Attend prenatal or parenting classes that
may provide contacts for lactation support.
4. Online Resources:

Consultant Websites: Many lactation consultants have
websites where you can learn about their services and book
appointments.
Telehealth Services: Some consultants offer virtual
consultations if in-person visits are not feasible.
4. What to Expect During a Consultation
1. Initial Assessment:

Health History: The consultant will review your and your
baby's health history and any specific concerns.
Observation: They will observe a feeding session to assess the
latch, positioning, and baby's feeding patterns.
2. Hands-On Guidance:

Techniques: They will demonstrate and help you practice
proper latching and positioning techniques.
Problem-Solving: Provide solutions and strategies to address
specific breastfeeding challenges.
3. Personalized Plan:

Feeding Plan: Develop a personalized feeding plan based on
your needs and goals.

Follow-Up: Schedule follow-up consultations to monitor progress and adjust the plan as needed.
4. Emotional Support:

Reassurance: Offer emotional support and encouragement to boost your confidence.
Resources: Provide additional resources such as educational materials and support group information.
Conclusion
Seeking the help of a lactation consultant can be invaluable in overcoming breastfeeding challenges and ensuring a successful breastfeeding journey. By understanding when and how to seek professional advice, you can address issues early, enhance your breastfeeding experience, and provide the best possible nutrition for your baby.

Partner and Family Support: Involving Your Loved Ones
1. The Importance of Support
1. Emotional Backing:

Boosts Confidence: A supportive partner and family can significantly boost a mother's confidence in her ability to breastfeed.
Reduces Stress: Emotional support helps reduce stress, which can positively impact milk production.
2. Practical Assistance:

Shared Responsibilities: Sharing household and baby care duties allows the mother to focus on breastfeeding.
Physical Support: Helping with tasks like diaper changes, burping, and soothing the baby can make a big difference.
3. Creating a Positive Environment:

Encouragement: Positive reinforcement and encouragement from loved ones can enhance the breastfeeding experience.

Comfort: A comfortable, stress-free environment is essential for successful breastfeeding.

2. Involving Your Partner

1. Educating Together:

Learn Together: Attend breastfeeding classes or read breastfeeding books together to understand the process and challenges.
Understand Benefits: Knowing the benefits of breastfeeding for both baby and mother can increase partner support.

2. Practical Support:

Night Feedings: Partners can bring the baby to the mother for night feedings and help with burping and changing.
Pumping Assistance: If the mother is pumping, the partner can assist with cleaning and preparing pumping equipment.

3. Emotional Support:

Listening Ear: Sometimes, just listening to the mother's concerns and experiences can be incredibly supportive.
Encouraging Words: Offer words of encouragement and appreciation for the mother's efforts and dedication.

3. Involving Other Family Members

1. Education and Awareness:

Inform Family: Educate other family members about the benefits of breastfeeding and the importance of support.
Set Expectations: Make sure family members understand and respect your breastfeeding goals and routines.

2. Practical Help:

Household Chores: Family members can help with cooking, cleaning, and other household chores to free up time for breastfeeding.

Babysitting: Offering to take care of older children can allow the mother to focus on breastfeeding the newborn.
3. Creating a Supportive Atmosphere:

Respect Privacy: Ensure that family members respect the mother's privacy and provide a comfortable space for breastfeeding.
Positive Reinforcement: Encourage family members to offer positive reinforcement and avoid criticism or unsolicited advice.
4. Building a Support Network
1. Support Groups:

Join Groups: Join local or online breastfeeding support groups where mothers can share experiences and advice.
Family Involvement: Partners and family members can also attend support group meetings to better understand the breastfeeding journey.
2. Professional Guidance:

Lactation Consultants: Seek advice from lactation consultants who can provide professional support and answer questions.
Healthcare Providers: Involve healthcare providers in discussing breastfeeding challenges and strategies with the family.
5. Communicating Effectively
1. Open Communication:

Express Needs: Encourage the mother to openly express her needs and concerns to her partner and family.
Active Listening: Family members should practice active listening and show empathy and understanding.
2. Setting Boundaries:

Clear Boundaries: Establish clear boundaries regarding breastfeeding practices and the level of involvement from family members.

Respect Decisions: Ensure that family members respect the mother's decisions and breastfeeding choices.

Conclusion

Involving your partner and family in your breastfeeding journey can provide crucial emotional and practical support, making the experience more positive and successful. By educating loved ones, sharing responsibilities, and fostering a supportive environment, you can create a strong network that benefits both you and your baby. Remember, effective communication and mutual understanding are key to building a supportive and empowering breastfeeding experience.

1. Triumph Over Challenges
Story 1: Sarah's Journey to Success

Background: Sarah, a first-time mother, faced initial difficulties with latching and low milk supply.
Challenges: Struggled with painful latching, frequent feeding sessions, and societal pressure to switch to formula.
Overcoming Obstacles: With the support of a lactation consultant and a dedicated breastfeeding support group, Sarah improved her baby's latch and boosted her milk supply through frequent pumping and skin-to-skin contact.
Success: Sarah successfully breastfed her baby for two years, sharing her story to inspire other mothers facing similar challenges.
Story 2: Emma's Return to Work

Background: Emma, a working mother, was determined to continue breastfeeding after returning to her demanding job.
Challenges: Balancing work responsibilities, finding time to pump, and maintaining milk supply.
Overcoming Obstacles: Emma created a pumping schedule, utilized her company's lactation room, and enlisted the support of her employer and colleagues.
Success: Emma managed to breastfeed exclusively for six months and continued partial breastfeeding for a year, proving that it is possible to balance career and breastfeeding.
2. Breastfeeding Twins and Multiples
Story 3: Laura's Tandem Nursing Experience

Background: Laura, a mother of twins, faced the unique challenge of breastfeeding two babies simultaneously.

Challenges: Coordinating feedings, managing exhaustion, and ensuring both babies received adequate nutrition.

Overcoming Obstacles: Laura used tandem nursing pillows, developed a feeding schedule, and received help from her partner and family to manage household tasks.

Success: Laura exclusively breastfed her twins for six months, continuing to breastfeed alongside introducing solids, demonstrating that breastfeeding twins is achievable with the right support and strategies.

Story 4: The Johnson Family's Triple Triumph

Background: The Johnsons welcomed triplets and were committed to breastfeeding despite the odds.

Challenges: The logistical complexity of feeding three babies, maintaining milk supply, and handling the physical and emotional demands.

Overcoming Obstacles: With guidance from a lactation consultant and an organized feeding and pumping schedule, the Johnsons found their rhythm.

Success: The triplets thrived on breast milk, and the family's story became a source of motivation for parents of multiples.

3. Overcoming Societal and Cultural Barriers

Story 5: Maria's Cultural Journey

Background: Maria, originally from a community where formula feeding was the norm, faced cultural resistance to breastfeeding.

Challenges: Lack of community support, misconceptions about breastfeeding, and pressure to conform to local practices.

Overcoming Obstacles: Maria educated herself on breastfeeding benefits, sought support from online communities, and found a local breastfeeding group.

Success: Maria exclusively breastfed her baby, becoming an advocate in her community and helping other mothers see the value of breastfeeding.

Story 6: Aisha's Advocacy

Background: Aisha, an immigrant in a country with different breastfeeding norms, struggled with integrating her breastfeeding journey into her new cultural environment.
Challenges: Language barriers, limited access to breastfeeding resources, and cultural differences.
Overcoming Obstacles: Aisha connected with multicultural breastfeeding support groups and used translation services to communicate with healthcare providers.
Success: Aisha successfully breastfed her baby and became a cultural ambassador, promoting breastfeeding awareness and support within her community.
4. Breastfeeding Preemies
Story 7: Grace's Preemie Miracle

Background: Grace gave birth to a premature baby who needed intensive care.
Challenges: Baby's inability to latch initially, reliance on pumping, and managing stress and fear.
Overcoming Obstacles: With the NICU's support, Grace began pumping immediately, provided expressed milk through a feeding tube, and practiced kangaroo care.
Success: Grace's baby gradually learned to latch, and she continued to breastfeed successfully after NICU discharge, emphasizing the power of persistence and love.
Story 8: David's NICU Journey

Background: David, a single father, faced the challenge of supporting his preemie's breastfeeding needs.
Challenges: Managing NICU visits, learning about lactation, and ensuring his baby received breast milk.
Overcoming Obstacles: David worked closely with NICU staff, used donor milk when necessary, and educated himself about breastfeeding.

Success: David's baby thrived, and he became a role model for other single parents navigating the breastfeeding journey.

5. Extended Breastfeeding

Story 9: Megan's Extended Journey

Background: Megan chose to breastfeed her child beyond infancy.

Challenges: Facing societal judgment, balancing extended breastfeeding with other dietary needs, and managing personal health.

Overcoming Obstacles: Megan joined extended breastfeeding support groups and educated her community about the benefits of long-term breastfeeding.

Success: Megan breastfed her child until the child naturally weaned, highlighting the importance of following one's intuition and the child's needs.

Story 10: Rachel's Tandem Nursing

Background: Rachel continued to breastfeed her toddler while nursing a newborn.

Challenges: Juggling the needs of two breastfeeding children, dealing with fatigue, and ensuring nutritional balance.

Overcoming Obstacles: Rachel received guidance from a lactation consultant and support from her partner and family.

Success: Rachel successfully tandem nursed, showing that extended breastfeeding and nursing siblings can be a rewarding experience.

Conclusion

These inspiring stories demonstrate that while breastfeeding comes with its challenges, it also brings immense joy and fulfillment. By sharing these journeys, this chapter aims to encourage, motivate, and provide hope to every mother on her breastfeeding path. Whether you face difficulties, societal pressures, or special circumstances, know that you are not alone and that success is within reach with determination, support, and love.

Real-Life Experiences: Stories from Breastfeeding Mothers

In this section, we delve into the real-life experiences of breastfeeding mothers who have navigated the joys and challenges of breastfeeding. Through their candid accounts, you'll gain insight, inspiration, and solidarity in your own breastfeeding journey. These stories highlight the diversity of experiences, the triumphs over obstacles, and the profound bond between mother and child forged through breastfeeding.

Story 1: Sarah's Journey
Sarah, a first-time mother, shares her journey of overcoming initial struggles with latching and low milk supply. Through perseverance and support, she successfully breastfed her baby, proving that determination can lead to breastfeeding success.
Story 2: Emma's Triumph

Emma, a working mother, shares her experience of balancing a demanding career with breastfeeding. Despite challenges, she found creative solutions and support systems that allowed her to continue breastfeeding her baby, showcasing the power of resilience.
Story 3: Laura's Twin Adventure
Laura, a mother of twins, recounts her unique journey of breastfeeding two babies simultaneously. With patience, dedication, and specialized techniques, she embraced the joys and challenges of tandem nursing, demonstrating the remarkable capabilities of the female body.
Story 4: Maria's Cultural Shift

Maria shares her story of navigating cultural barriers and misconceptions surrounding breastfeeding in her community. Through education, advocacy, and perseverance, she challenged societal norms and empowered herself and other mothers to embrace breastfeeding.
Story 5: Grace's Preemie Miracle

Grace reflects on her experience of breastfeeding her premature baby in the NICU. Despite the initial hurdles, she found strength in the bond with her baby and the support of healthcare professionals, illustrating the resilience of both mother and child.
Story 6: Megan's Extended Journey

Megan shares her decision to breastfeed her child beyond infancy, despite societal judgment. Through her journey of extended breastfeeding, she celebrates the enduring connection and nourishment it provides, inspiring other mothers to follow their instincts.
Story 7: Rachel's Tandem Nursing

Rachel opens up about her experience of tandem nursing her toddler and newborn, embracing the challenges and joys of nurturing two children simultaneously. Her story underscores the profound bond and emotional fulfillment that breastfeeding brings to both mother and child.
Through these heartfelt narratives, we honor the diverse experiences and journeys of breastfeeding mothers everywhere, celebrating their strength, resilience, and unwavering commitment to nurturing their babies with love and nourishment.

Overcoming Adversity: How Others Have Faced and Overcome Challenges

In this section, we explore the resilience and determination of breastfeeding mothers who have confronted and conquered various obstacles on their breastfeeding journeys. From physical difficulties to societal pressures, these stories illustrate the power of perseverance, support, and belief in the benefits of breastfeeding.

Story 1: Lily's Physical Hurdles

Lily shares her journey of overcoming physical challenges such as inverted nipples and mastitis. Through perseverance and seeking professional guidance, she was able to overcome these obstacles and establish a successful breastfeeding relationship with her baby.

Story 2: Emily's Mental Health Struggles

Emily opens up about her battle with postpartum depression and how it impacted her breastfeeding experience. With the support of her healthcare provider and loved ones, she sought help and found solace in breastfeeding, which became a source of comfort and healing.

Story 3: Sofia's Cultural Barriers

Sofia recounts her experience of breastfeeding in a culture where formula feeding is predominant. Despite facing criticism and pressure to conform, she remained steadfast in her decision to breastfeed, advocating for herself and educating others about the benefits of breastfeeding.

Story 4: Aiden's Tongue Tie Challenge

Aiden's mother shares their journey of discovering and addressing his tongue tie, which initially hindered breastfeeding. Through persistence, consultation with lactation professionals, and undergoing a simple procedure, Aiden was able to latch properly, and breastfeeding became a joyful experience for both mother and baby.

Story 5: Mia's Return to Work

Mia navigates the challenges of returning to work while continuing to breastfeed her baby. Despite initial anxieties about maintaining milk supply and finding time to pump, she developed a supportive routine with her employer and colleagues, ensuring a smooth transition and continued breastfeeding success.
Story 6: Isabella's Journey with Twins

Isabella shares her experience of breastfeeding twins, acknowledging the unique challenges of tandem nursing and managing the demands of two infants. Through determination, patience, and support from her partner and healthcare professionals, she successfully nourished her twins with breast milk, highlighting the strength of maternal love. These stories of resilience and triumph inspire and empower breastfeeding mothers to persevere through challenges, seek support when needed, and embrace the transformative journey of nurturing their babies with breast milk. By sharing their experiences, these mothers offer hope, encouragement, and solidarity to others facing similar obstacles on their breastfeeding paths.

Celebrating Success: The Joys of Breastfeeding

In this section, we celebrate the profound joys and transformative experiences that breastfeeding brings to mothers and babies alike. Through heartwarming anecdotes and reflections, these stories capture the beauty, intimacy, and sheer delight of the breastfeeding journey.

Story 1: Emma's Bonding Miracle
Emma shares the profound bond she forged with her baby through breastfeeding. As she cradled her little one close, she felt a deep connection and overwhelming sense of love, experiencing moments of pure joy and contentment that only breastfeeding could provide.
Story 2: Ava's Milestone Moments

Ava reminisces about the precious milestones she witnessed while breastfeeding her baby. From the first fluttering kicks during nursing sessions to the adorable coos and smiles exchanged between mother and child, each moment served as a reminder of the magical bond they shared.
Story 3: Ethan's Comfort and Security

Ethan's mother recounts the comfort and security he found in breastfeeding during challenging times. Whether soothing him during teething pains or comforting him during illness, breastfeeding became a source of solace and reassurance for both mother and baby.
Story 4: Lily's Empowerment Journey

Lily reflects on the empowerment she felt as she nourished her baby through breastfeeding. Despite initial doubts and insecurities, she embraced her body's ability to provide for her child, finding strength and confidence in the intimate act of nursing.
Story 5: Noah's Developmental Delights

Noah's mother marvels at the developmental milestones her baby achieved through breastfeeding. From the robust growth and thriving health to the cognitive leaps and bounds, breastfeeding played a vital role in nurturing his overall well-being and development.

Story 6: Harper's Unbreakable Bond

Harper's mother cherishes the unbreakable bond she shares with her baby through breastfeeding. As they gazed into each other's eyes during nursing sessions, they communicated love, trust, and an unspoken connection that transcended words. These stories serve as a testament to the immeasurable joys and blessings of breastfeeding, from the tender moments of bonding to the profound sense of fulfillment and empowerment it brings to mothers and babies alike. By celebrating these moments of joy and connection, we honor the beauty and significance of the breastfeeding journey for generations to come.

Conclusion: Your Breastfeeding Journey Ahead

As you reach the conclusion of this book, you stand at the threshold of a remarkable journey — the journey of breastfeeding. Throughout these pages, you've gained insights, wisdom, and guidance to embark on this transformative path with confidence and conviction. But beyond the words on these pages lies the real adventure — the adventure of nurturing your baby, forging an unbreakable bond, and experiencing the profound joys of motherhood.

Your breastfeeding journey is unique, filled with ups and downs, triumphs and challenges, but know that you're not alone. You join a community of mothers worldwide, united by the shared experience of nourishing their babies with love and devotion. As you navigate this journey, remember these words:

Embrace the journey: Embrace the journey: Embrace the journey with an open heart and an open mind. Embrace the moments of connection, the tender snuggles, and the quiet whispers exchanged during nursing sessions. Embrace the challenges as opportunities for growth and learning, knowing that every hurdle overcome strengthens your resolve and deepens your bond with your baby.

Trust your instincts: Trust your instincts: Trust your instincts as a mother. You possess an innate wisdom that guides you in nurturing and caring for your baby. Listen to your intuition, follow your instincts, and trust in the incredible capabilities of your body to provide for your little one's needs.

Seek support: Seek support: Seek support from your loved ones, healthcare providers, and fellow breastfeeding mothers. Surround yourself with a supportive network that uplifts and encourages you on your breastfeeding journey. Whether you need advice, reassurance, or simply a listening ear, know that you're not alone.

Celebrate every milestone: Celebrate every milestone, no matter how small. Celebrate the first latch, the first smile, and the first time your baby gazes up at you with eyes full of love and trust. Celebrate the precious moments of connection and intimacy that breastfeeding brings into your life, cherishing each one as a gift.

Above all, remember that your breastfeeding journey is a testament to the love, dedication, and nurturing spirit that define motherhood. As you continue on this journey, may you find strength in your own resilience, joy in the moments shared with your baby, and fulfillment in the profound bond you share. Your breastfeeding journey is a beautiful, transformative experience — one that will forever shape and enrich your life and the life of your precious little one.

So, as you embark on this extraordinary adventure, may you embrace each day with gratitude, courage, and an unwavering commitment to nurturing your baby with love, tenderness, and the timeless gift of breast milk. Your breastfeeding journey awaits — embrace it with open arms and an open heart.

Reflecting on Your Experience: Looking Back and Moving
Forward

As you conclude your journey through the pages of this book,
take a moment to reflect on the experience you've gained and
the insights you've gathered along the way. Your journey into
the world of breastfeeding has been filled with discovery,
learning, and growth, and now, as you prepare to move
forward, it's essential to pause and acknowledge how far
you've come.

Reflect on your journey: Reflect on the challenges you've faced
and the triumphs you've celebrated. Remember the moments
of doubt and uncertainty, and recognize the strength and
resilience that carried you through. Reflect on the bonds
you've forged with your baby, the joys you've experienced,
and the profound love that fuels your commitment to
breastfeeding.

Acknowledge your growth: Acknowledge the growth you've
experienced as a mother and as a breastfeeding advocate.
Recognize the newfound confidence you've gained in your
ability to nurture and nourish your baby. Celebrate the
knowledge you've acquired and the skills you've honed,
knowing that each step forward brings you closer to achieving
your breastfeeding goals.

Honor your journey: Honor your journey for its uniqueness
and its significance in shaping the mother you've become.
Embrace the lessons learned, the wisdom gained, and the
memories created along the way. Whether your breastfeeding
journey has been smooth sailing or marked by obstacles, know
that every experience has contributed to your growth and
your bond with your baby.

Embrace the future: Embrace the future with hope, optimism, and a sense of purpose. As you look ahead to the days and weeks to come, envision the possibilities that lie before you. Trust in your instincts, draw upon your newfound knowledge, and continue to nurture your baby with love, compassion, and dedication.

Remember, your breastfeeding journey is not just a chapter in a book—it's a lifelong commitment to the health and well-being of your baby. As you move forward, may you carry with you the lessons learned, the memories cherished, and the bonds strengthened through the beautiful journey of breastfeeding.

With each passing day, may you find renewed joy, fulfillment, and connection in the act of breastfeeding, knowing that you are providing your baby with the most precious gift of all—your love, your care, and the nourishment of breast milk. Embrace your journey, embrace your role as a breastfeeding mother, and embrace the boundless possibilities that lie ahead.

Encouragement and Empowerment: Trusting Your Instincts

Dear Reader,

As you prepare to embark on the remarkable journey of breastfeeding, I want to offer you words of encouragement and empowerment. In this wondrous adventure, amidst the tender moments and the inevitable challenges, one of your greatest allies will be your own intuition.

Trust in your instincts, for they are the gentle whispers of wisdom guiding you along this path. From the moment you cradle your baby in your arms, you possess an innate knowing—a deep connection that transcends words. Listen to this inner voice, for it will lead you with grace and certainty.

Believe in the power of your body, for it is a marvel of nature. Within you flows the life-giving sustenance that nourishes your precious little one. Trust in the miraculous ability of your breasts to provide exactly what your baby needs, exactly when they need it.
Embrace each moment with confidence, knowing that you are uniquely equipped to meet the challenges that may arise. While advice and guidance are valuable, remember that you are the expert on your baby. Your instincts are finely attuned to their needs, offering comfort, nourishment, and reassurance.

In moments of doubt or uncertainty, draw strength from the knowledge that you are not alone. Reach out to fellow mothers, lactation consultants, and supportive communities. Share your experiences, seek wisdom, and find solace in the collective wisdom of those who have walked this path before you.

Above all, trust in the bond that you share with your baby. It is a bond forged in love, nurtured through the gentle rhythm of breastfeeding. In the quiet moments of connection, in the soft sounds of suckling, you will find the profound beauty of motherhood.

So, dear reader, as you embark on this sacred journey, trust in your instincts. They are your compass, your guiding light, leading you ever closer to the boundless love and joy that await you on the path of breastfeeding.

With warmth and encouragement,
Queen Wilz
 Final Words: Continued Support and Resources for Your
Breastfeeding Journey

Dear Reader,

As you reach the end of this book, know that your journey
into the world of breastfeeding is just beginning. While these
pages have provided guidance, insight, and encouragement,
your path forward is illuminated by the unwavering support
and resources available to you.

In the days, weeks, and months ahead, may you find comfort
in knowing that you are not alone on this journey. Seek out
the support of fellow mothers, lactation consultants, and
breastfeeding advocates who can offer guidance, wisdom, and
reassurance along the way.
Explore the wealth of resources available to you, from online
communities and support groups to reputable websites,
books, and professional organizations. Arm yourself with
knowledge, empower yourself with information, and trust in
your ability to navigate the joys and challenges of
breastfeeding.

Remember, every breastfeeding journey is unique, and there is
no one-size-fits-all approach. Trust in your instincts, listen to
your baby, and embrace the beauty of the bond that unfolds
between you.

Above all, be gentle with yourself. Motherhood is a journey of
learning, growth, and transformation, and it is okay to seek
help and support when you need it. Your well-being matters
just as much as your baby's, so prioritize self-care and
compassion as you embark on this sacred journey.

As you continue on your breastfeeding journey, may you find joy in the moments of connection, strength in the challenges overcome, and love in the bond shared with your precious little one.

With warmest wishes for continued success and fulfillment,

Queen Wilz.